Facilitating Hearing and Listening in Young Children

Second Edition

Early Childhood Intervention Series

Series Editor
M. Jeanne Wilcox, Ph.D.

Facilitating Hearing and Listening in Young Children, Second Edition by Carol Flexer, Ph.D.

Working with Parents of Young Children with Disabilities by Elizabeth J. Webster, Ph.D., and Louise M. Ward, M.A.

Pediatric Swallowing and Feeding: Assessment and Management edited by Joan C. Arvedson, Ph.D., and Linda Brodsky, M.D.

Premature Infants and Their Families by M. Virginia Wyly, Ph.D.

A Practical Guide to Family-Centered Early Intervention by P. J. McWilliam, Ph.D., Pamela J. Winton, Ph.D., and Elizabeth Crais, Ph.D.

Facilitating Hearing and Listening in Young Children

Second Edition

■

Carol Flexer, Ph.D.
The University of Akron

Singular Publishing Group, Inc.
San Diego · London

Singular Publishing Group
401 West A Street, Suite 325
San Diego, California 92101-7904

Singular Publishing Group, Inc., publishes textbooks, clinical manuals, clinical reference books, journals, videos, and multimedia materials on speech-language pathology, audiology, otorhinolaryngology, special education, early childhood, aging, occupational therapy, physical therapy, rehabilitation, counseling, mental health, and voice. For your convenience, our entire catalog can be accessed on our web-site at **http//www.singpub.com**. Our mission to provide you with materials to meet the daily challenges of the everchanging health care/educational environment will remain on course if we are in touch with you. In that spirit, we welcome your feedback on our products. Please telephone **(1-800-521-8545)**, fax **(1-800-774-8398)**, or e-mail (**singpub@singpub.com**) your comments and requests to us.

© 1999 by Singular Publishing Group, Inc.

Typeset in 10/12 New Century Schoolbook by SoCal Graphics

Printed in the United States of America by BookCrafters
Second Printing October 1999

Library of Congress Cataloging-in-Publication Data

Flexer, Carol Ann.
    Facilitating hearing and listening in young children / Carol
Flexer. — 2nd ed.
       p.   cm. — (Early childhood intervention series)
    Includes bibliographical references and index.
    ISBN 1-56593-989-1 (softcover : alk. paper)
    1. Hearing disorders in children.   2. Hearing disorders in
infants.   3. Hearing impaired children—Rehabilitation. I. Title.
II. Series
    [DNLM: 1. Hearing Disorders—in infancy & childhood.
2. Rehabilitation of Hearing Impaired—in infancy & childhood. WV
271 F619f 1999]
RF291.5.C45F54   1999
618.92'0978—dc21
DNLM/DLC
for Library of Congress

93-42099
CIP

Contents

■

Foreword

■

When current social policy regarding infants and young children who are at-risk is considered in conjunction with advances in theoretical conceptualization and associated research, it is clear that early childhood intervention is emerging as a unique and dynamic area of scientific inquiry across multiple disciplines. The purpose of the Early Childhood Intervention Series is to provide state-of-the-art information with respect to interventions focusing on families and their infants and young children who are at risk for or have diagnosed disabilities. As readers will readily recognize, this is no small task; the "art" of effective intervention practices is continually subject to refinement and improvements in existing practices as well as the introduction of entirely new ideas and approaches. As is the case with most topics subject to a rapid surge in scholarly attention, new findings and ideas are often steps ahead of their practical application and, in some cases, are not easily translated into appropriate practices, creating what many have come to regard as a science-practice gap. Books in this series have been designed and prepared with an eye toward reducing this gap and assisting early childhood intervention personnel in becoming consumers of current theoretical and empirical information. The topics in the series are wide ranging and, through explicit examples and discussion in each of the individual books, offer a wealth of practical information to assist us all in providing the most effective interventions for families and their infants and young children.

The present volume is the second edition of *Facilitating Hearing and Listening in Young Children*. In this new edition, the author integrates recent scientific advances in amplification technology, child development, and auditory neuroscience to generate a highly readable and updated resource. The book continues the author's primary focus on educational audiology and provides a wealth of practical ideas for maximizing children's hearing and listening across a broad base of early intervention program types and activities. Families, teachers, early interventionists, speech-language pathologists, and audiologists will find this book an invaluable addition to their bookshelves.

M. Jeanne Wilcox, Ph.D.
Series Editor

Preface

■

The second edition of *Facilitating Hearing and Listening in Young Children* continues the author's desire to promote the awareness and use, in early intervention programming, of hearing as the initial and primary receptive/input modality for communication and learning for all young children. Due to today's incredible amplification technology, opportunities for early identification and intervention, and increased knowledge of brain function and child development, the nature of auditory stimulation of the brain has assumed monumental proportions.

The information in this book certainly is appropriate and applicable for use in programming for children with any degree of hearing impairment. Focusing on hearing and listening is equally appropriate for young children with normal hearing sensitivity. If an infant or young child cannot hear clearly, intervention that uses spoken communication to impart information will be minimally effective. In other words, the sensory input modality of hearing must be facilitated to create an optimal learning environment for infants and young children with disabilities. Accordingly, this book maintains the orientation toward maximizing (a) the hearing sensitivity of children, (b) the listening and learning environments of children at home and in early intervention programs, and (c) the integrity and redundancy of the speech signal.

This book has been written with an educational focus, and is intended for primary use by early intervention educational personnel, including parents, teachers, speech-language pathologists, audiologists, and classroom assistants. It is designed for audiologists who are interested in providing more detailed management recommendations for acoustic accessibility. The focus for speech-language pathologists, teachers, classroom assistants, and parents is on featuring auditory-based learning strategies and on becoming informed consumers of audiological services.

Primary topics include the many facets of hearing and hearing impairment, the critical role of hearing in one's life, the structure and function of the ear, and types and degrees of hearing impairment, with special emphasis on otitis media, behavioral and objective (electrophysiological) measurement of hearing, technological management of hearing, and facilitation of listening skills. New information has been added about amplification technology, cochlear implants, federal laws, and listening strategies.

Information in this book is presented in a practical, no-nonsense fashion, with summary checklists provided at the end of each chapter. Reader-friendly fact sheets detail various types of hearing technologies, including hearing aids, personal FM units, sound-field FM (classroom) amplification systems, and mild gain hard-wired units. There also are guidelines for maximizing hearing and the auditory environment, with suggestions for hearing management strategies that may be included in the Individualized Family Service Plan or the Individualized Educational Plan as mandated by federal laws. Specific strategies for the development of listening skills are detailed, and an extensive glossary of terms used by audiologists is provided at the end of the book.

The intention of this second edition is to emphasize the need and strategies for creating an *auditory world* for children. This book is not about "auditory training," it is about "auditory living." Hearing is not a small unrelated piece of language and life for children. Rather constant, meaningful "listening" stimulation of young children's critical auditory brain centers develops their neurological and experiential foundations for literacy and learning. This book provides a vision for auditory management and listening development that will propel us into the next century.

Acknowledgments

■

The second edition of *Facilitating Hearing and Listening in Young Children* was inspired by many friends, family members, and colleagues. Thanks to my husband Pete, my children, and my mother for their patient encouragement. I would like to extend a special thank you to Catherine Richards, M.A., for her assistance in writing Chapters 6 and 7. Catherine is an audiologist and speech-language pathologist at Hudson Schools in Hudson, Ohio.

Dedication

■

This book is dedicated to my children: Heather, Hillari, and David; to my grandchildren: Yehuda, Rachel, and Yishai; and to the many infants and children who experience auditory disorders. All deserve an opportunity to hear and listen.

■ CHAPTER 1
The Importance of Hearing and the Impact of Hearing Problems

INTRODUCTION

Recent census data show that, while 82% of Americans, overall, complete high school (Manning, 1998), 43% of the students in special education programs do not (Boutte, 1998). Approximately 27% of the population in the United States has a bachelor's degree. The more education a person has, the more pay they are likely to earn: People without a high school diploma earn an average of $15,011 per year; with a high school diploma, $22,154; with a bachelor's degree, $38,112; and with an advanced degree, $61,317 per year (Manning, 1998).

So what? After all, this book is about early intervention, not about preparing for college. The fact is, the neurological foundations that we foster during the first critical years of a child's life provide the "velcro" for the attachment of later linguistic, literary, and academic competencies (Gilbertson & Bramlett, 1998; Sharpe, 1994). Therefore, it is possible that, in many instances, when a child is unable to graduate from high school, it is because we unintentionally diluted a powerful ingredient for brain integrity—audition.

Studies in brain development show that sensory stimulation of the auditory centers of the brain is critically important, and indeed, influences the actual organization of auditory brain pathways (Boothroyd, 1997; Chermak & Musiek, 1997; Musiek & Berge, 1998).

The same brain areas—the primary and secondary auditory areas—are most active when a child listens and when a child reads. That is, phonological or phonemic awareness, which is the explicit awareness of the speech SOUND structure of language units, forms the basis for the development of reading skills (Gilbertson & Bramlett, 1998).

The point is, anything that we can do to "program" those critical and powerful auditory centers of the brain with acoustic detail will expand children's opportunities.

Now, consider how the following situations, observed in early intervention programs, obscure the detection of detailed and precise auditory signals, with subsequent deprivation of the auditory centers of the brain. Will these children have the opportunity to develop their auditory neurological foundations for language, reading, and learning?

1. Sally, age 18 months, has Down syndrome. She appears unresponsive to her environment and inattentive to speech. Permanent hearing impairment had been ruled out by electrophysiologic tests; however, she has the stenotic (abnormally small) ear canals and chronic ear infections typical of 88% of children with Down syndrome (Strome, 1981). She is receiving medical management but continues to experience chronic hearing loss due to ear wax and middle ear fluid. Her spoken communication skills are far below her expected cognitive potential, yet her hearing sensitivity, the listening environment, and the speech signal are not being managed. Sally does not use any hearing technologies, the acoustic environment has not been controlled, and listening skills have not been developed.

2. Johnny was born almost 3 months prematurely. He does not have a diagnosed hearing loss. At 20 months, he is receiving language facilitation at home due to receptive and expressive language delay. On a typical day in his home, the television is blaring, traffic noises enter from the street, and Johnny's mother speaks to him from across the room. Johnny appears unaware of his mother's speech and does not seem to be making progress in the acquisition of language skills. Johnny must have access to a clear, complete, and highly redundant and meaningful speech signal if he is to have an opportunity to develop spoken communication skills. Therefore, his listening and learning environment needs to be as quiet as possible, and the speaker must be close to him (in the absence of assistive listening devices).

3. There are six children in a developmental preschool classroom. Five have histories of continual ear infections, all have docu-

mented attention problems, and all have moderate-to-severe language delays. None of the children has been diagnosed as hearing impaired; thus none of the children is receiving any audiologic or educational management for their hearing difficulties. The classroom is rather large with a tile floor and a high, cement ceiling. There is a constant roar from the heating system, and the gym next door is in continual use. Four different activities are occurring simultaneously, causing a high noise level in the classroom. Sound measurements show that, at any given point in the classroom, noise levels are louder than speech levels. Ironically, these six children, who need a quiet and focused learning environment, have virtually no access to spoken instruction!

Certainly no one intended to sabotage the learning opportunities of the children in the previous examples. The problem is that hearing and listening are so ambiguous and elusive. Furthermore, there is no good substitute for hearing. If there was, hearing problems would pose no unique educational dilemmas. Hearing impairment of any type and degree is problematic (Bess, 1985; Northern & Downs, 1991). Even a slight hearing impairment can interrupt a child's language-learning process and interfere with his or her development. Hence, assessment and management of a child's hearing sensitivity and listening ability are pivotal to all educational programming that uses speech as the means of communication. Said another way, if a child cannot hear speech sounds clearly, or if a child does not have the skills to listen, or if the learning environment does not allow instruction to be heard clearly, any testing or intervention (including occupational therapy, physical therapy, psychological assessment, speech-language therapy) that uses speech as the vehicle for interaction is likely to fall far short of its projected goals. Therefore, an infant or child's hearing sensitivity and listening ability, and the quality of the learning environment, cannot be ignored or assumed; they must be known and optimized.

The purpose of this introductory chapter is to sensitize the reader to the invisible yet critical role of the sensory input modality of **hearing**. Topics covered include a discussion of the acoustic filter effect of hearing impairment, the role of hearing in life, a checklist of auditory behaviors as a function of developmental level, prevalence of hearing impairment in infancy and childhood, and a summary page of important points about hearing and hearing impairment.

■ WHAT IS HEARING IMPAIRMENT?

A primary reason why comprehensive and ongoing audiologic diagnostic *and management* services are not available in many early intervention programs is because many professionals have not been provided with basic knowledge about the critical role hearing plays in the developmental and educational processes (Lass et al., 1986; Luckner, 1991; Martin, Bernstein, Daly, & Cody, 1988; Ross, 1991). If the primacy of hearing is not understood, suggestions for hearing management may seem superfluous to a child's developmental progress.

It is important to recognize that children are not small adults. Children bring a different "listening" to a communicative/learning situation than do adults, in two main ways. First, human auditory brain structure is not fully mature until about age 15 years; thus, a child does not bring a complete neurological system to a listening situation (Boothroyd, 1997; Chermak & Musiek, 1997). Second, children do not have the years of language and life experience that enable adults to fill in the gaps of missed or inferred information (such filling-in of gaps is called auditory/cognitive closure). Therefore, children require more complete, detailed auditory information than adults.

Hearing and listening form the invisible cornerstones of spoken communication. Infants and toddlers spend much of their day engaged in active or passive listening activities as a means of obtaining information from their environments. The need for all children to be able to hear clearly must not be underestimated (Berg, Blair, & Benson, 1996).

Word-Sound Distinctions

The importance of children learning to discriminate word-sound distinctions was documented by Elliott, Hammer, and Scholl (1989). They administered several tests to children who had normal hearing sensitivity and found that the ability to perform fine-grained auditory discrimination tasks (e.g., to hear "ba" and "pa" as distinctly different syllables) correctly classified nearly 80% of the primary-level children in their study either as progressing normally or having language and learning difficulties. The authors concluded that auditory discrimination skills are associated with the development of basic academic competencies that are essential for successful educational performance. If a child cannot hear phonetic distinctions as early as his or her first year of life, he or she is at significant risk for language learning problems (Leonard, 1991) and for later academic failure (Ross, 1991).

The ability to discriminate the word-sound distinctions of individual phonemes or speech sounds is defined as *intelligibility*. The ability simply to detect the presence of speech is defined as *audibility*. If, because of a hearing impairment, noisy environments (homes, cars, outdoors, classrooms, stores, zoos, and preschools are examples of typical environments that can be too noisy if not controlled), or poor attending and listening skills, an infant or toddler cannot discriminate *feet* from *eat*, for example, he or she will not learn appropriate semantic distinctions unless deliberate intervention occurs.

The Invisible Acoustic Filter Effect of Hearing Impairment

The importance of hearing to the communication and learning processes tends to be significantly underestimated because *hearing impairment is invisible*; thus the effects of hearing impairment often are associated with problems or causes other than hearing impairment (Davis, 1990; Ross, 1991). For example, when a toddler responds inappropriately to requests (e.g., brings his mom a toy *boat* when his mom asked for his *coat*), or when an infant or toddler does not seem "connected" to his or her environment, the cause of the child's behaviors may be attributed to noncompliance or to slow learning rather than to hearing impairment. Furthermore, when an infant or toddler has a diagnosed developmental disability and delayed behaviors are expected, the confounding impact of hearing impairment often is totally overlooked.

The ambiguity of hearing impairment is further magnified by the tendency to erroneously categorize hearing impairment into only two classifications: normal hearing or deafness (Ross & Calvert, 1984). Such dichotomous thinking rules out the necessity of considering hearing in early intervention programming. That is, an infant or toddler who is diagnosed as deaf is believed to be able to hear nothing, whereas the other alternative is normal hearing in which case hearing management strategies are thought to be unnecessary.

A child with a fluctuating hearing impairment, unilateral hearing impairment, or mild to moderate hearing impairment obviously is not deaf. It is important to note that about 94 to 96% of people with hearing impairment are functionally hard of hearing rather than deaf (Ross & Calvert, 1984). The concept that hearing impairment occurs along a broad continuum needs to be emphasized as does the fact that very few people have no hearing at all.

Any type and degree of hearing impairment can present a significant barrier to an infant or child's ability to receive information from the environment (Bess, 1985; Cargill & Flexer, 1989; Davis, 1990; Flexer, Wray, & Ireland, 1989; Northern & Downs, 1991; Ross, Brackett, & Maxon, 1991).

Early intervention personnel may have difficulty understanding how even a slight hearing impairment can have such a detrimental influence on language and development. Hearing impairment is nothing more than an invisible acoustic filter that distorts, smears, or eliminates incoming sounds (Davis, 1990; Ling, 1989) (see Figure 1–1). The detrimental effects of this acoustic filter cause the difficulty. The primary negative effect of the invisible acoustic filter of hearing impairment is its impact on verbal language acquisition. If a child has a prelingual severe or profound hearing impairment, the child will not learn to speak unless intensive intervention occurs (Ling, 1989). If speech sounds are not clearly detected due to a more moderate hearing impairment or a continuously fluctuating hearing impairment, a child's spoken language probably will not be clear either, *unless* deliberate intervention occurs (Ling, 1989). We speak because we hear, and we speak *what* we hear.

The secondary negative consequence of the invisible acoustic filter effect of hearing impairment is its destructive impact on the

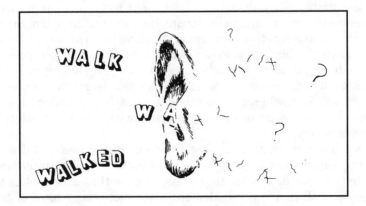

Figure 1–1. Hearing impairment acts like an invisible acoustic filter that distorts, smears, or eliminates incoming sound. (Illustration by Jackie Rios)

higher level linguistic skills of reading and writing (Ross, 1990; Wray, Hazlett, & Flexer, 1988). If a child cannot hear clearly enough to identify word-sound distinctions, then discrete verbal language concepts probably will not develop spontaneously. If verbal language skills are spotty or deficient, reading skills also are likely to be deficient because reading is a secondary linguistic function built on speaking (Simon, 1985). To continue with the concept of the snowballing negative consequences of hearing impairment, if a child has poor reading skills, his or her academic options will be limited because literacy is linked to academics (Gilbertson & Bramlett, 1998) (see Figure 1–2).

The cause of this unfortunate chain of events is that ambiguous, invisible, underestimated, and ignored acoustic filter effect of hearing impairment. Relative to early intervention, the core problem of hearing impairment must be recognized and hearing must be accessed to **prevent** problems at the secondary levels of spoken language development, reading, and academics (Davis, 1990; Ling, 1989; Ross & Giolas, 1978).

It is critical to reemphasize that human beings are neurologically wired to develop spoken language and reading skills through the central auditory system. Most people think that reading is a visual skill. But recent research on brain mapping shows that the primary reading centers of the brain are located in the auditory cortex—the auditory portions of the brain (Chermak & Musiek, 1997). Thus, children who are born with hearing loss and lack access to complete auditory input at a young age (through strong hearing aids or a cochlear implant and auditory-based teaching) tend to have a great deal of difficulty reading, even if their vision is normal. The earlier and more efficiently we can provide access to meaningful and detailed sound, with subsequent direction of the child's attention to sound, the better opportunity he or she will have to develop spoken language, literacy, and academic skills. **With the technology and early auditory intervention available today, a child with a hearing loss *can* have the same opportunity as a typical child to develop spoken language, reading, and academic skills through the auditory, and not the visual, channel**.

Early intervention personnel often misinterpret the cause of an infant or toddler's behaviors that result from the invisible acoustic filter effect of hearing impairment because the *barrier* to reception of clear and intelligible speech imposed by a hearing impairment typically is not identified (Ross, 1991). Speech might be audible to a child with a hearing impairment, but the words

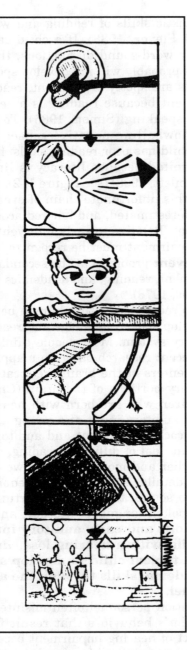

Figure 1–2. Unmanaged hearing impairment has a negative impact on the development of spoken communication, written communication, academics, professional options, and independent functioning. (Illustration by Josh Klynn)

may not be intelligible without technological intervention, especially in less than ideal acoustic environments (i.e., noisy settings). For example, a toddler with a mild hearing impairment might hear *eat, feet, beeped, she,* and *sleeps,* all as *ee.* All of the words might sound alike to the child but each conveys a different meaning. If the infant or toddler could be asked if he or she could hear the parent or therapist, the child's response likely would be "yes." How could a young and linguistically naive child understand that the high intensity vowel sounds and suprasegmental structures of the utterances are audible, but the high-frequency, low-energy morphological markers for place, tense, and plurality are not acoustically distinguishable?

Thus, it is common for early intervention personnel to make statements such as, "Of course Bobby has a bit of a hearing impairment. But hearing impairment is the least of his problems. His primary problem is that he has such poor oral expressive behavior." Perhaps Bobby's limited oral expressive behavior is caused wholly, or in part, by the acoustic filter effect of his hearing impairment. Until Bobby's hearing is accessed through assistive technology and he is taught to listen for crucial word-sound distinctions, he may have limited success improving his spoken language skills. The point is, the sensory modality of hearing cannot be ignored or bypassed in the schemata of intervention, just as the roots of a tree cannot be ignored if fruit is expected to grow.

Computer Analogy

One way to illustrate the potentially negative effects of any type and degree of hearing impairment on a child's language and overall development is to use a computer analogy. The primary concept is: **Data input precedes data processing**.

An infant or toddler (or anyone) must have information/data in order to learn. A primary avenue for entering information into the brain is through the ears via hearing (Lennenberg, 1967; Leonard, 1991). If data are entered inaccurately, incompletely, or inconsistently, analogous to using a malfunctioning computer keyboard or to having one's fingers on the wrong keys of a computer keyboard, the child will have incorrect or incomplete information to process. How can a child be expected to learn when the information that reaches his or her brain is deficient? (See Figure 1–3.) Is it the brain's fault that the data entered are incomplete? Is the computer program in error if the keyboard entry is faulty? Unfortunately, children who have inaccurate data entry may be labeled

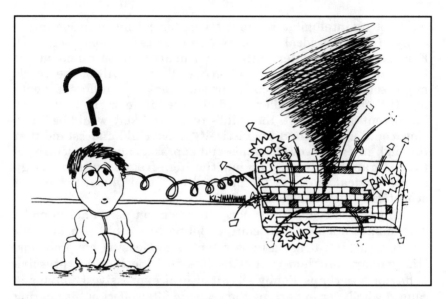

Figure 1–3. Hearing impairment is analogous to having a malfunctioning computer keyboard that interferes with data entry to the brain. (Illustration by Josh Klynn)

learning disabled, attention disordered, hyperactive, or noncompliant, because they behave in that fashion due to inaccurate, incomplete, and inconsistent data entry.

To continue the computer analogy, once the keyboard is repaired or the figurative fingers are placed on the correct keys of the keyboard allowing data to be entered accurately, analogous to using amplification technology that enables a child to detect word-sound distinctions, what happens to all of the previously entered inaccurate and incomplete information? (See Figure 1–4). Is there a magic button that automatically converts inaccurate data to complete and correct information? Unfortunately, all of the corrected data need to be reentered. Thus, the longer a child's hearing problem remains unrecognized and unmanaged, the more destructive and far-reaching are the snowballing effects of hearing impairment (see Figure 1–5).

Hearing is only the **first** step in the chain of intervention. Once hearing has been accessed as much as possible through appropriate signal-to-noise ratio enhancing technology, the child will have an opportunity to discriminate word-sound distinctions as a basis for learning language, which in turn provides the child with an opportunity to communicate and acquire knowledge of the

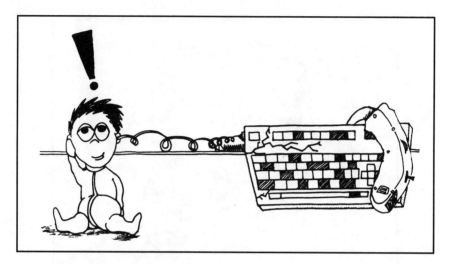

Figure 1–4. Amplification technology facilitates data entry by providing a more accessible keyboard. (Illustration by Josh Klynn)

world. All levels of the acoustic filter effect of hearing impairment need to be understood and managed.

The longer a child's data entry is inaccurate, the more damaging the snowballing acoustic filter effects will be on the child's overall life development. Conversely, the more intelligible and complete the data entered are, the better opportunity the infant or toddler will have to learn language which serves as a foundation for later reading and academic skills.

The point is, from the inception of early intervention programming, comprehensive audiologic and hearing management is an absolutely necessary first step for a child of any age with any type of hearing or listening difficulty to have an opportunity to learn.

A critical caveat is that, although amplification technology can provide a better "keyboard," a more efficient and consistent route of data entry, that keyboard will not be perfect. Thus, listening and learning strategies also need to be implemented.

■ THE ROLE OF HEARING

Hearing plays a vital and often subtle role in our lives, a role that must be understood to appreciate the impact of hearing impairment and the benefits of hearing management strategies. The functions of

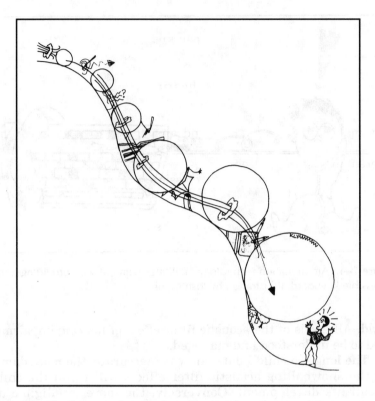

Figure 1–5. The longer a hearing impairment of any type and degree remains unrecognized and unmanaged, the more destructive are the snowballing effects of hearing impairment on the development of communication skills, learning, and functioning. (Illustration by Josh Klynn)

hearing can be divided, roughly, into three levels: primitive, signal warning, and spoken communication (Davis & Silverman, 1978).

Primitive Level

The most unconscious function of hearing is the primitive level which carries the auditory background, sounds that serve to identify a location. A hospital sounds different than a school which sounds different than a department store. Typically, we do not think about these sounds; however, if a location does not sound as expected, we become uneasy. If you have ever entered an empty hospital or an empty school, you have probably felt a bit anxious.

Biological sounds also are heard at the primitive level. Sounds like breathing, swallowing, chewing, heart beat, and pulse furnish proof that we are indeed alive and functioning. People who suddenly lose their hearing have been known to experience acute psychosis due to feelings of disconnectedness with the environment, time, and their own bodies.

Less dramatically, a new hearing aid or assistive listening device alters the wearer's auditory background by amplifying sounds previously not heard. This change in auditory background may make a wearer nervous and anxious without understanding why. Certainly, a baby or young child cannot explain that an altered auditory background may be a factor causing him or her to resist amplification. Yet, as professionals, we should be sensitive to the fact that there often is an adjustment period to amplification (typically, at least 1 month), due in part to the user's altered auditory background. One also could speculate about the effects of a constantly fluctuating hearing impairment like otitis media (ear infections) on a child's auditory background.

Signal Warning Level and Passive Learning

Signal warning, the second level of hearing function, is less subtle and pertains to monitoring the environment. Hearing and vision are distance senses, which allow us to know what is happening away from our bodies. However, we do not always have to see to know what is occurring. A baby in bed at night hears people talking, the television prattle, a typewriter's clatter, dogs barking, cars roaring, and so on. Knowing what is going on around us promotes feelings of security, whereas not knowing induces anxiety.

Unfortunately, persons with hearing impairment of any degree, even when wearing suitable hearing aids, cannot hear well over distances (see Figure 1–6). Distance hearing is problematic because the speech signal loses both intensity and critical speech elements as the signal travels away from the sound source (Leavitt & Flexer, 1991). The greater the hearing impairment, the greater the reduction in **earshot or distance hearing** (Ling, 1989). Said another way, the greater the hearing impairment or listening problem, the closer the listener must be to the speaker in order for speech to be heard at levels loud enough and with sufficient redundancy to be understood.

A child with a hearing impairment, even a mild or a unilateral impairment (hearing impairment in one ear; the other ear is normal), cannot casually overhear what people are saying or the events that are occurring (Davis, 1990). Children with normal hearing often seem to passively absorb information from the environment and to constantly have out little antennae to pick up

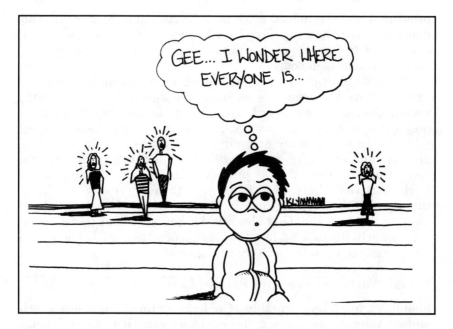

Figure 1–6. Persons with hearing impairment cannot hear well over distances, which disrupts the environmental monitoring function of hearing and often causes feelings of isolation. (Illustration by Josh Klynn)

every morsel of information. A child who has a hearing problem may seem oblivious to environmental events, "out of it," not to know what is occurring, unconnected to his or her environment, or have to be told everything.

Because of the reduction in signal intensity and integrity with distance, a child with a hearing problem may have a limited range or distance of hearing; that child may need to be taught directly many skills that other children learn incidentally.

Without being mindful of a reduction in speech intensity and information with increasing distance, a professional can confuse audibility and intelligibility (Boothroyd, 1978, 1984). A child may appear to hear and behave as if sounds are audible. However, sounds that are audible are not necessarily intelligible. A child may respond in a seemingly appropriate way, but actually be responding to the intonation patterns rather than to the specifics of an utterance (Boothroyd, 1978, 1984). A child with a hearing impairment might hear other people speaking, even from a distance, but not be able to hear one speech sound as distinct from another. Words like "walk, walked, walks," and "walking" could be indistinguishable; and words like "invitation" and "vacation" might be confused (Bess, 1985; Dobie & Berlin, 1979). Word confusions such as these have a strong potential for limiting a child's concept and vocabulary development.

Further implications of reduction of distance hearing include lack of access to the redundancy of spoken information that occurs in day-to-day transactions and lack of access to social cues (Conway, 1990). Much information children learn is not directed to the child, yet this tangential information is important for them to learn. Children learn how to start a conversation, request, problem solve, negotiate, compromise, joke, tease, and use sarcasm by "listening-in" to the conversation of others. For example, a family reported that their young child, who was later found to be moderately hard of hearing, would constantly take food from the kitchen without asking permission. This behavior was viewed by the family as disruptive to the family's function and the child was thought to be weird and noncompliant. Once the hearing impairment was identified and managed, the family recognized that the child had observed his siblings getting food from the kitchen, but he had never overheard them asking the parents for permission. Once the family realized that this child needed to be taught directly the family social behavior that the other children had learned passively, the child's behavior improved dramatically.

Beware of underestimating the barrier that any type and degree of hearing impairment presents to the casual acquisition of information from the environment (Ross, 1991) (see Figure 1–7).

Spoken Communication

The most obvious effect of the acoustic filter phenomenon discussed previously is on the development of spoken communication. Speech develops naturally because we hear. If an infant or child does not hear well, spoken communication does not develop well, or naturally.

Further, it takes a great deal of hearing and active listening before verbal language begins to take form (Ling, 1989; Northern & Downs, 1991; Pollack, 1985; Ross & Calvert, 1984; Vaughn, 1981). A normal, hearing child does not begin to use discernible words until approximately 1 year of age, after months of meaningful, interactive, listening. In fact, because the inner ear is fully

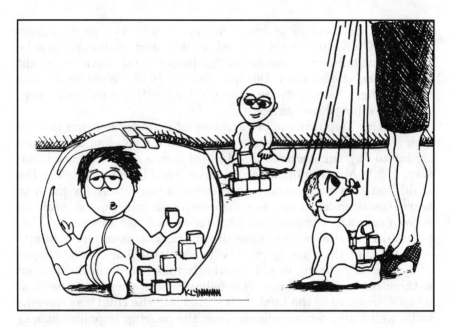

Figure 1–7. Hearing impairment of any type and degree is a barrier to incidental learning. (Illustration by Josh Klynn)

developed by the fifth month of gestation, an infant with normal hearing potentially has had 4 months of in utero auditory stimulation prior to birth (Northern & Downs, 1991). Thus, a great deal of listening input does, and indeed must, occur (about 16 months) before verbal output can be expected.

The point is, if a child has a hearing impairment, even a mild one, those many months of listening must be recouped; listening time cannot be skipped (Cole & Gregory, 1986). The brain must still be programmed with accurate verbal input before verbal ouput can occur.

Listening time commences when hearing is accessed, typically through amplification. For example, if a child with a hearing impairment is 2 years old chronologically when amplification begins, he or she is only 1 day old in listening age—clearly, another strong argument for early intervention (Ling, 1989; Ross & Calvert, 1984; Rowe, 1985). When that same child reaches a chronological age of 4 years, he or she now has a listening or hearing age of 2 years. That is, this child has had 2 years' experience in hearing detailed spoken language and receiving auditory information from the environment. Therefore, we would expect this child to have spoken language skills closer to those of a 2-year-old child than to those of a 4 year old. With active and thoughtful auditory intervention, this gap between hearing age and chronological age is expected to diminish. Hence, the younger a child is when he or she receives the necessary amplification technology, the less time a gap between hearing age and chronological age will exist.

■ CHECKLIST OF AUDITORY BEHAVIORS AS A FUNCTION OF DEVELOPMENTAL LEVEL

As discussed previously, hearing impairment can be manifested in ambiguous ways. Nevertheless, there are some obvious behaviors that a child with normal hearing should display. Following is a checklist of auditory behaviors as a function of developmental àge (Hayes & Northern, 1996). Note, however, that any child who experiences developmental disabilities is at risk for hearing impairment and listening difficulties and thus may need repeated audiologic evaluations.

Checklist of Auditory Behaviors

Caution: Be sure that visual and tactile cues do not contaminate auditory responses.

Birth to 3 months. If sleeping quietly, infant awakens to sudden noises; cries to sudden, very loud sounds; startles or jumps to sudden, loud sounds; is soothed by mother's voice; gurgles, coos, and laughs.

3 to 6 months. Turns eyes and head to search for the location of sound, responds to mother's voice, makes a large variety of babbling sounds and imitates "oohs and ba-bas," changes voice pitch, enjoys rattles and other sound-making toys, appears "connected" to the environment (i.e., seems aware of surroundings and notices people and events).

6 to 10 months. Turns to and attempts to find sounds outside of visual field; responds to own name, telephone ringing and someone's voice, even when not loud; understands "no," "bye-bye," and other common words; and makes sounds with rising and falling inflections and listens to music or singing.

10 to 15 months. Turns to find a sound behind him or her, demonstrating the ability to respond to sounds at a significant distance (distance hearing); imitates simple sounds and words; produces a large variety of different sounds including vowels and consonants; jabbers in response to human voice; can point to or look at familiar objects or people when asked to do so; shows evidence of being able to acquire information passively (i.e., the child can learn from events that are not directed actively to him or her).

15 to 18 months. Can hear and respond when called from another room; voice sounds normal; first words are well on their way; can follow simple spoken directions without visual (pointing or eye gaze) or tactile cues; identifies people, body parts, and toys on request; gestures with speech appropriately; bounces in rhythm with music; repeats some words that you say.

■ PREVALENCE OF HEARING IMPAIRMENT

Audiologic services in early intervention and school programs typically have been viewed as *support services*, relevant for only a very small population of children who are labeled as deaf (Blair, 1986; Brackett, 1992). Although children diagnosed as deaf certainly require audiologic services, the necessity for hearing management is **not** limited to these few children.

There are approximately 40 million school children in the United States, and at least 7 million of them have some degree of hearing impairment (Berg, 1986a; Davis, 1990; Niskar et al., 1998; Ross, Brackett, & Maxon, 1991). Consequently, when a persistent minimal, mild, or moderate hearing impairment (thresholds worse than 15 dB HL) is recognized for the disabling condition it is (Bess, 1985; Dobie & Berlin, 1979; Northern & Downs, 1991), children with hearing impairment represent the largest single population of school children requiring special services (Niskar et al., 1998). According to the American Speech-Language-Hearing Association (ASHA) recommendation of one educational audiologist for every 12,000 school children (ASHA, 1993), we would need at least 3,333 additional audiologists to provide the full spectrum of audiologic services in schools in the United States. The 750 audiologists currently employed full-time in the schools are able to manage less than 1% of the children who need support for mainstreamed placement; they certainly are too few in number to manage even a fraction of the infants and toddlers who are eligible for early intervention services under Public Law 99-457 (Education of the Handicapped Act Amendments of 1986).

Upfold (1988) reported that the population of children with hearing impairment has changed over the past decades. Specifically, there are fewer children with severe-to-profound hearing impairment, because of the virtual elimination of maternal rubella and Rh incompatibility, and many more children with mild-to-moderate hearing impairment who have been identified and fitted with amplification. Surprisingly, the number of children with severe-to-profound hearing impairment is half that known 10 years ago (Upfold, 1988).

The actual incidence of minimal, mild, and moderate hearing impairment, most often caused by otitis media with effusion (middle ear infections), may be much higher than school screenings lead us to believe (Anderson, 1991; Ross, 1991). Hearing screening environments in schools typically have less than ideal levels of ambient noise; therefore, hearing tends to be screened at 20 to 35 dB HL (Anderson, 1991). As a consequence of environmental conditions, school screenings may miss many children who are at risk for academic failure because even a 15 dB hearing impairment poses a significant problem for the young child who must learn crucial word-sound distinctions (Dobie & Berlin, 1979; Northern & Downs, 1991).

Lundeen (1991) conducted a prevalence study in which he tested the hearing of 38,000 school children. Unfortunately, Lundeen's data can be misleading because he used the criterion of a pure-tone average of greater than 25 dB HL as constituting hearing impairment. This criterion is at least 10 dB higher than that known to pose educational and learning problems. Lundeen found that only 2.63% of the children from grades 1 to 12 and 5.51% of first graders had pure-tone averages greater than 25 dB HL.

When 15 dB HL is used as the criterion for identifying an educationally significant hearing impairment, the incidence increases dramatically. In fact, the Third National Health and Nutrition Examination Survey found that 14.9% of the 6,166 school children tested (ages 6–19 years) had low-frequency or high-frequency hearing loss of at least 16 dB (Niskar et al., 1998). In another study conducted in the Putnam County, Ohio, school district, it was found that, in the *primary grades*, 43% of the students failed a 15 dB HL hearing screening on any given day and about 75% of the primary-level children in a class for children with learning disabilities failed a 15 dB HL hearing screening (Flexer, 1989).

Another study, the MARRS (Mainstream Amplification Resource Room Study, National Diffusion Network Project) study on sound-field (classroom) amplification found that about 30% of the children in grades 3 through 6 and 75% of the children in primary-level classes for children with learning disabilities failed a 15 dB hearing screen (Ray, Sarff, & Glassford, 1984). In yet another study, Flexer, Millin, and Brown (1990) were surprised to discover that only one of the nine children with developmental disabilities in their study of classroom amplification had thresholds of 15 dB HL or better when tested in a sound-isolated booth; none of the children they tested had been identified by the school as having hearing difficulties.

The point is, the incidence of developmentally and educationally significant hearing impairment may be underestimated tremendously, and many of the infants, toddlers, and children with fluctuating or minimal hearing impairments will not be identified by hearing screenings. Indeed, the words "mild" and "minimal" should be avoided because such terminology implies *without consequence*.

A minimal or slight hearing impairment (greater than 15 dB HL) may not be problematic for a linguistically mature person who has sophisticated and disciplined attending skills and is able to share meaning with the speaker; but a minimal hearing impairment can sabotage the overall development of an infant or child who is in the process of learning language and acquiring knowledge (Davis, 1990; Downs, 1988).

Unfortunately, many schools and early intervention programs continue to use the educational models that might have been appropriate for the population of children with hearing impairment that existed 10 to 50 years ago: children with severe-to-profound hearing impairments who were identified rather late and did not have access to early intervention services (McGee, 1990; Ross & Calvert, 1984). Schools often act as if all the children who require special services for hearing impairment are deaf. If the children are not labeled as deaf, they are believed to not require services (Davis, 1990; Ross, 1991). Today's large population of children who are hard of hearing is a very different population than the population that existed decades ago, and they often can be accommodated through progressive hearing management in mainstreamed settings (Brackett, 1997; McGee, 1990).

■ CHECKLIST OF IMPORTANT POINTS ABOUT HEARING AND HEARING IMPAIRMENT

☐ Auditory stimulation is necessary for the development of critical auditory brain centers.

☐ Hearing and listening form the invisible cornerstones of the language/learning system.

☐ Hearing impairment occurs along a broad continuum ranging from a slight hearing loss to a profound hearing impairment; not as two discrete groupings of normally hearing or deaf. In fact, 94 to 96% of persons with hearing impairment are hard of hearing and not deaf.

☐ Hearing impairment, whether slight or profound in nature, if unmanaged, has a negative impact on the development of spoken language communication, reading, writing, and academic competencies.

☐ Human beings are neurologically wired to develop spoken language and reading skills primarily through the central auditory system.

☐ Speech may be audible to someone with a hearing impairment but not necessarily intelligible enough to hear one word as distinct from another.

☐ Hearing is a primary way that information is entered into the brain; data input precedes data processing.

☐ Any type and degree of hearing problem can present a significant barrier to the child's ability to receive information from the environment.

☐ Hearing impairment of any degree causes a reduction in earshot or distance hearing that interferes with a child's ability to benefit from passive learning; the speech signal may not be loud enough or clear enough for the child with a hearing problem if the speaker is not very close to the listener.

☐ Children with hearing impairments need to be taught, directly, many concepts, vocabulary, and social/emotional cues that children with normal hearing learn incidentally.

☐ The population of children with hearing impairment is shifting. Today, the number of children with severe-to-profound hearing impairment is less than half what it was 10 to 30 years ago due to the reduction in maternal rubella and Rh incompatibility. There are many more children with mild-to-moderate hearing impairments who have been identified and fitted with amplification.

☐ A slight or mild hearing loss (greater than 15 dB HL but less than 40 dB HL) may not be problematic for a linguistically mature person who has sophisticated and disciplined attending skills; but a minimal hearing impairment can seriously affect the overall development of an infant or child who is in the process of learning language, developing spoken communication skills, and acquiring knowledge.

■ CHAPTER 2

Structure and Function of the Ear

■ DEFINING SOUND

To understand the causes of hearing impairment, it is first important to gain an appreciation for the intricate, complex, but incredibly tiny mechanism called the ear. Even though the human ear does not look very impressive from the outside, its range of sensitivity to sound, from the softest sound that can just barely be detected to one that is uncomfortably loud, is 10,000,000 to 1 (Stach, 1998). In fact, the average human ear is so sensitive that it can almost detect random molecular movement.

When sound is heard, the individual actually is interpreting a pattern of vibrations that originate from a source in the environment. Sound waves in the air, produced by the movement or vibration of air molecules, are analogous to the water waves produced when a pebble is thrown into a pond. Just as the pebble causes ripples to emanate from the point at which the pebble entered the pond, sound waves also start at the point where sound is generated and spread out in circles of waves.

The sound waves that we hear are vibrational energy, and they travel through the air at a speed of about one fifth of a mile per second; 1,130 feet per second. The simplest form of sound wave is called a sine wave, simple harmonic motion. A sine wave (see Figure 2–1), heard as a pure tone, can be graphed as a circle on a flat plane plot.

Sound has both physical and psychological characteristics. The physical dimensions of speech sounds are frequency, intensity, and

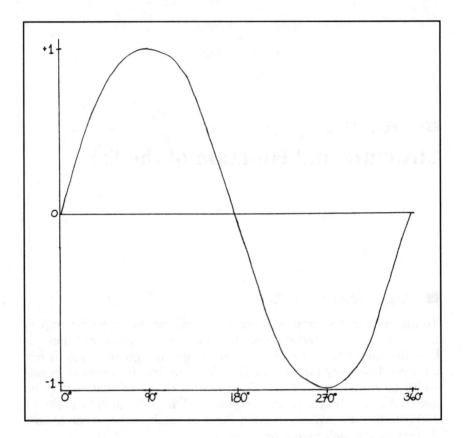

Figure 2–1. A sine wave, which is a circle (360°) graphed on a flat plane plot, is the simplest form of sound; it is heard as a pure tone. (Illustration by Josh Klynn)

duration. The product of these three characteristics defines our ability to perceive sound, and a hearing impairment may affect the perception of one or all of these features.

Pitch and loudness are psychological attributes of sound. The physical parameter of frequency corresponds to the psychological attribute of pitch. High-frequency sounds are perceived by the listener to be high in pitch, whereas low-frequency sounds are perceived to be low in pitch. Loudness is the psychological correlate of the physical parameter of intensity. The more intense the sound, the louder it is perceived.

One is reminded of the riddle, "If a tree fell in the forest and no one was around, would a sound still be made by the falling tree?" The answer depends on whether one is describing sound from a physical or a psychological basis. The physical parameters of intensity, frequency, and duration exist independent of an observer, but the psychological perception of loudness, pitch, and time requires the presence of a person.

Frequency refers to the number of back-and-forth oscillations or cycles produced by a sound source in a given time period. Hertz (Hz) and cycles per second (cps) are terms used to describe frequency. The frequency of the sound is measured by counting the number of cycles per second of the sound wave. One cycle equals the distance between the top (crest) of one sound wave and the top of the next sound wave. If a vibrator or sound source was set into motion and completed 1,000 back-and-forth cycles in 1 second, it would have a frequency of 1000 Hz. Fewer cycles per second characterize low frequencies, whereas many cycles per second typify high frequencies. As seen in Figure 2–2, as the frequency of the sound increases, wavelengths become shorter and the number of cycles per second increases.

Humans are able to hear frequencies ranging from 20 to 20,000 Hz; however, frequencies between 250 and 4000 Hz are particularly important for the perception of speech. Low-pitched sounds, with frequencies of 500 Hz and below, have a bass quality. Relative to speech sounds, low-pitched sounds carry the melody of speech, vowel sounds, and most environmental sounds (Ling, 1989). Importantly, 90% of the energy of speech is carried in the lower frequencies (see Table 2–1).

High-pitched sounds, on the other hand, have frequencies above 1500 Hz and have a tenor quality. High-frequency sounds are very important for hearing speech because they carry the energy involved in consonant production. That is, high frequencies carry the meaning of speech, whereas low frequencies, primarily, carry the melody. Only 10% of the energy of speech but 90% of the meaning is carried by the higher frequencies. One is not aware of the higher pitch components of speech sounds because the fundamental frequency of vocal fold vibration overrides the higher formant frequencies and is all that is consciously heard.

There is approximately a 30 dB range between the softest and most powerful speech sounds throughout the frequency range. The weakest, least intense speech sound is /Θ/ as in thin. The strongest, most intense speech sound is /a/ as in law.

Intensity of sound is defined as pressure or power. Intensity is measured in decibels (dB) and graphed as amplitude on a sine wave (see Figure 2–3). The intensity of a sound is determined by

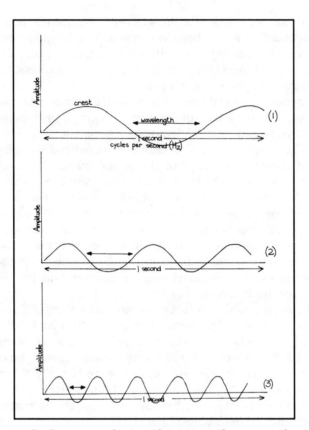

Figure 2–2. As the frequency of a sound increases (from examples 1 to 3), the wavelengths become shorter, the number of cycles per second (Hz) increases, and the sound is perceived as becoming higher in pitch. (Illustration by Josh Klynn)

the degree of displacement of air particles that occurs as a sound is made. Intensity involves the strength of sound waves traveling from the sound source. The abbreviation dB stands for decibel; the B is capitalized in honor of Alexander Graham Bell. The softest sound a typical young adult with normal hearing can just barely detect is defined as 0 dB hearing level (HL). The loudness of a person whispering a few feet away is about 25 to 30 dB HL. The average loudness of typical conversational speech in a quiet environment when the speaker is a few feet away is 45 to 50 dB HL. An alarm clock is about 80 dB HL, city traffic is about 70 dB HL, a

TABLE 2–1. Speech Information Available at 250 Hz, 500 Hz, 1000 Hz, 2000 Hz, 4000 Hz (Adapted from Ling, 1989; 1997)

At 250 Hz, plus or minus 1/2 octave, the following speech information is available:
1st Formant of vowels /u/ and /i/
The Fundamental Frequency of females' and childrens' voices
Male voice harmonics
Voicing cues
Suprasegmental patterns (stress, rate, inflection, intonation); prosody
Nasal murmur associated with m, n, ng

At 500 Hz, plus or minus 1/2 octave, the following speech information is available:
1st Formants of *most* of the vowels
Harmonics of *all* voices (male, female, child)
Voicing cues
Nasality cues
Suprasegmentals
Some plosive bursts associated with /b/ and /d/

At 1000 Hz, plus or minus 1/2 octave, the following speech information is available:
2nd Formants of back and central vowels
Important CV and VC transition information
Nasality cues
Some plosive bursts
Voicing cues
Suprasegmentals
Unstressed morphemes
The important acoustic cues for *manner* of articulation are available at 1000 Hz

At 2000 Hz, plus or minus 1/2 octave, the following speech information is available:
THIS IS THE KEY FREQUENCY FOR INTELLIGIBILITY OF SPEECH
The important acoustic cues for *PLACE* of articulation are available at 2000 Hz
2nd and 3rd Formant information for front vowels
CV and VC transition information
Acoustic information for the liquids /r/ and /l/
Plosive bursts
Affricate bursts
Fricative turbulence

At 4000 Hz, plus or minus 1/2 octave, the following speech information is available:
This is the key frequency for /s/ and /z/ morpheme audibility. The /s/ and /z/ phonemes are critical for language learning because they signal:

plurals	idioms	possessives	auxiliaries
3rd person	questions	copulas	past perfect

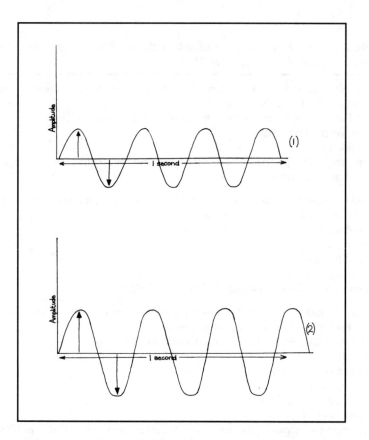

Figure 2–3. Intensity is determined by the degree of displacement of air particles that occurs as a sound is made, and is graphed as amplitude on a sine wave; the increase in amplitude from examples 1 to 2 represents an increase in intensity that is perceived as an increase in loudness. (Illustration by Josh Klynn)

food blender is about 90 dB HL, a rock concert can be louder than 110 dB HL, a jet airport can have sounds as intense as 120 dB HL, and a firecracker has a bang at about 140 dB HL (Berg, 1993).

The decibel is a logarithmic and not a linear scale, which means that every dB counts a great deal. For example, if a sound increases or decreases 10 times in intensity, the change is only 10 dB. A 20 dB change means that a sound is 10×10, or 100 times as intense as the original sound. To use an example, the average hearing impairment caused by ear infections is 20 dB and is labeled a slight or minimal hearing impairment. When one understands that the dB scale is logarithmic, it is recognized that in reality, this "slight" hearing impairment means that the child hears approximately 10 times less well when the infection is present as he or she can hear when the fluid is cleared.

Most sounds in our environment are complex in structure. Complex sounds are comprised of many frequencies with varying intensities occurring at the same time (see Figure 2–4). Speech is an example of complex sound.

In all learning domains—home, school, and community settings—there are a variety of sounds from many sources. Sounds that are desirable can be called acoustic signals, whereas undesirable sounds typically are referred to as noise. Noise levels tend to

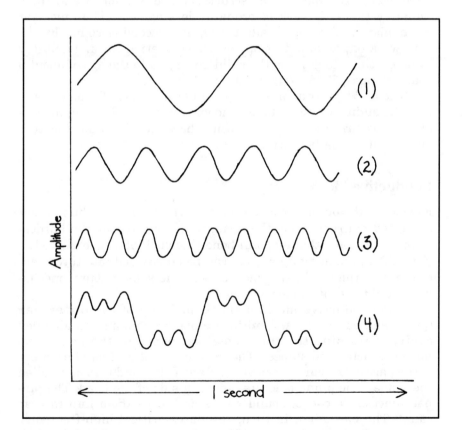

Figure 2–4. Complex sounds are made up of many frequencies with varying intensities occurring at the same time; example 4 is a complex wave formed by the combination of the pure tones represented in examples 1, 2, and 3. (Illustration by Josh Klynn)

be more intense in the low frequencies, and then the intensity fades and become less powerful at the higher frequencies. The weaker consonant sounds (i.e., th, s, sh, f, p) are affected by noise more rapidly than the vowel sounds. In noisy situations, the intelligibility of speech (the ability to hear word-sound distinctions clearly) is compromised even though the sounds might still be audible.

■ ANATOMY OF THE EAR

At birth, the auditory system of a child with normal hearing is functioning and completely developed (Northern & Downs, 1991). Specifically, the middle ear structures are developed and functional by the 37th week of prenatal development. The inner ear mechanism is developed, adult size, and receiving sound by the 20th week of prenatal development. The external ear and auditory canal continue to grow as the child grows, up to the age of about 9 years (Pappas, 1998; Wright, 1997).

The auditory system is an incredible structure. To understand how the auditory system breaks down resulting in hearing impairment, it is first necessary to discuss how the ear is put together and how it normally functions.

Conductive Mechanism

Except for the outer ear or pinna, the structure of the human ear is located entirely inside the head, well protected by the hardest bone in the body, the temporal bone (Stach, 1998). As observed in Figure 2–5, the auditory system can be subdivided into three general areas: the conductive mechanism, the sensorineural mechanism, and the central mechanism.

The conductive mechanism is made up of the **outer ear** (pinna and ear canal) and **middle ear** (eardrum and an air-filled cavity containing the three smallest bones in the body—the malleus, incus, and stapes). The most external portion of each ear is the part of the ear we can see, a flap of skin and cartilage called the pinna. One pinna is located on each side of the head. The pinnae function to collect sound waves and focus them into the ear canal. The ear canal, in turn, resonates critical high-frequency components of speech sounds. The resonant frequency of the typical ear canal is 2700 Hz, a crucial frequency for consonant intelligibility. Due to the presence of small hairs and ear wax, the ear canal also protects the delicate tympanic membrane (eardrum)

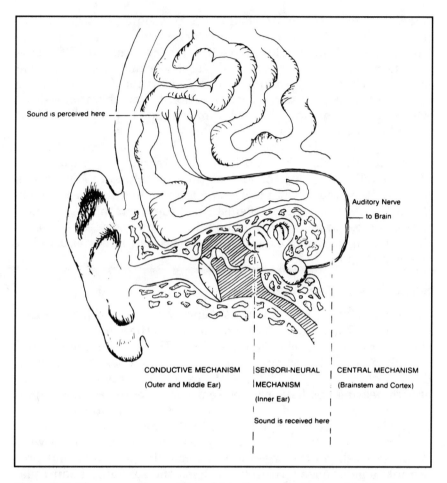

Sound is perceived here

Auditory Nerve
to Brain

CONDUCTIVE MECHANISM | SENSORI-NEURAL | CENTRAL MECHANISM
(Outer and Middle Ear) | MECHANISM | (Brainstem and Cortex)
(Inner Ear)

Sound is received here

Figure 2–5. The ear can be partitioned into the conductive mechanism, the sensorineural mechanism, and the central auditory system. (Illustration by Jackie Rios)

from debris. The eardrum is located at the end of the inside portion of the ear canal (see Figure 2–5). The eardrum is nearly horizontal in its position in the ear canal at birth, causing it to be difficult to view; it doesn't reach its more vertical position of 50–60 degrees from horizontal until the third year of life (Wright, 1997). It is the boundary between the outer and middle portions of the ear.

Sound waves entering the ear canal strike the eardrum, causing it to vibrate. These vibrations are conducted to the inner ear through the middle ear by the three smallest bones in the body, called the ossicles. These bones, the malleus, incus, and stapes, are interconnected and are attached to the tympanic membrane and a membrane called the oval window which serves as the gateway to the inner ear. The middle ear itself is a very small, air-filled cavity. Its primary function is to efficiently transmit the airborne sound hitting the eardrum to the fluid-filled inner ear. The eardrum vibrates, passing that vibration to the chain of ossicles which then pumps this vibrational information to the oval window, a window to the inner ear.

Air gets into the middle ear through the Eustachian tube, a small tube that runs from the back of the throat to the front wall of the middle ear cavity. As long as the Eustachian tube functions appropriately, the air that is used by the middle ear structures for metabolism is constantly replenished. If the Eustachian tube does not open often to allow air into the middle ear, disease can develop due to lack of sufficient oxygen. These diseases will be discussed in the next chapter.

Sensorineural Mechanism

The sensorineural mechanism is composed of the cochlea (**inner ear**) and VIIIth cranial nerve. The cochlea is the sensory portion of the sensorineural mechanism and the VIIIth cranial nerve is the neural portion. The general framework of the inner ear is housed deep inside the temporal bone of the skull and contains the organs of both hearing and balance. The sense organ of the ear is a highly specialized organ called the organ of Corti. It is contained within the cochlea, which is a small, coiled tube that has approximately 2½ turns and is about 3.5 cm long. The inner ear is filled with fluid. Hair cells in the organ of Corti contain stereocilia that project into a gelatinous structure overlying the specialized hair cells; the hair cells are the sensory receptors. Vibrational movements from the ossicles initiate a wave complex in the cochlear fluids that displaces the inner ear fluid and hair cells. The hair cells are the sensory receptors that change the hydraulic movement of the inner ear fluids into electrical impulses. The electrical impulses from the hair cells trigger nerve impulses in the auditory nerve. The auditory nerve, in turn, transmits the neural impulses to the many auditory centers of the brainstem and brain.

The inner ear also contains the vestibular or balance system. It is not unusual for an infant or toddler to have both a hearing and a balance disorder because the organs for vestibular and auditory detection are housed together in the inner ear.

Central Mechanism

The brainstem and cortex which comprise the central portion of the auditory system contain millions of complex patterns of neural connections. Sound enters the system through approximately 16,500 hair cells in the cochlea, is transmitted to about 30,000 neurons in the auditory nerve, and ultimately is processed by more than 200 million neurons in the brain.

Learning about the meaning of incoming sounds occurs in the central auditory system. Available neurological data suggest that, while myelination of the auditory nerve and brainstem are mostly complete by around 6 months of age, radiations from the brainstem to the auditory cortex continue until around 5 years of age and myelinations from the corpus callosum through the auditory cortex continue to develop until 15 to 20 years of age (Boothroyd, 1997). Therefore, even though infants have superior speech processing abilities by 6 months, there is a considerable period of development before these processing abilities reach adultlike levels.

■ THE PERIPHERAL-CENTRAL DISTINCTION

The outer, middle, and inner ear, together, are known as the **peripheral auditory system** and function to receive sounds from the environment. The central auditory system, located in the brainstem and auditory cortex, takes the sounds that have been fed in through the peripheral system and codes them for more complex, higher level auditory processes.

Thus, there are two general processes in hearing: (a) getting sounds to the brain through the outer, middle, and inner ear; and (b) learning the meaning of those sounds once they are in the brain. Obviously, sound must first be heard before learning can take place, just like computer data input must precede data manipulation.

Without sensory evidence (sound input), there can be no auditory perception (Boothroyd, 1997). Sensory evidence depends NOT only on the integrity of the peripheral mechanism, but also on the interactions between peripheral and central mechanisms; experience can play a major role in the development of that interaction (Boothroyd, 1997). Listening experience will be covered in more detail in Chapter 7.

CHAPTER 3

Types, Degrees, and Causes of Hearing Loss

■ INTRODUCTION

Infants and children must have access to detailed sound before auditory learning can occur. Hearing impairments from disease or damage in the auditory system interfere with sound access, thereby precluding, or certainly diluting, a child's auditory learning capabilities. **Sensory input and auditory experience are necessary for neural development and organization of the auditory brain centers**.

There are three general types of peripheral hearing impairments that interfere with sound access. Based on the location of the damage (the site of lesion) in the auditory system, hearing impairments may be classified as conductive, sensorineural, or mixed (Northern, 1996) (see Figure 3-1).

This chapter presents an overview of the general classifications of hearing impairment and then details specific pathologies that can cause hearing impairment in children. A list of factors that place an infant and child at risk for hearing impairment is included at the end of the chapter.

■ GENERAL CLASSIFICATIONS OF HEARING IMPAIRMENT

Time of Onset

Hearing impairments in children can be classified into congenital and acquired hearing losses relative to when in the child's life the

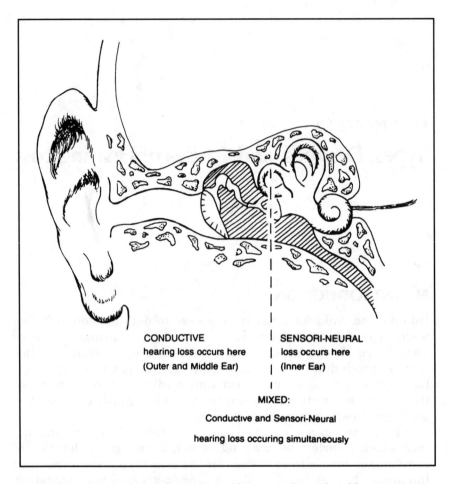

CONDUCTIVE
hearing loss occurs here
(Outer and Middle Ear)

SENSORI-NEURAL
loss occurs here
(Inner Ear)

MIXED:

Conductive and Sensori-Neural

hearing loss occuring simultaneously

Figure 3–1. There are three general classifications of peripheral hearing impairment based on site of lesion, or the location of damage within the ear: conductive, sensorineural, and mixed which is both conductive and sensorineural. (Illustration by Jackie Rios)

hearing impairment first occurs. *Congenital hearing impairments* typically occur before, at, or shortly after birth but prior to the learning of speech and language, usually before age 3 (Jacobson, 1997).

In contrast, *acquired hearing impairments* occur after speech and language have developed. The negative effects of an acquired hearing impairment tend to be less severe than those of a congenital hearing impairment because auditory brain centers have already been programmed for language and spoken communication.

The earlier a hearing impairment occurs in the developmental process, the more the hearing impairment interferes with language, learning, and enrichment of auditory brain function, unless the child receives effective intervention. A later occurring hearing impairment certainly requires intervention, but the consequences of an acquired hearing impairment are not as pervasive if the child already has established a relatively sophisticated linguistic system and rich neural connections in the auditory correx. An acquired hearing loss is still subject to the negative consequences of the acoustic filter phenomenon discussed in Chapter 1. Moreover, a child's speech can degenerate if the hearing loss is severe in degree and speech conservation therapy is not provided.

General Causes of Hearing Impairments

Both congenital and acquired hearing impairments can be caused by *endogenous* or *exogenous* factors (Fritsch & Sommer, 1991). Endogenous hearing impairments are genetic or hereditary. Hereditary hearing impairments have different probabilities of occurrence. For example, if a hearing impairment is genetically dominant, a single parent may carry the gene and each child has a 50% chance of receiving the gene and resultant hearing impairment. If the hearing impairment is genetically recessive, both parents must carry the gene and each child has a 25% probability of receiving both genes with resultant hearing impairment. A *multifactoral inheritance* means that there are additive effects of several minor gene-pair abnormalities in association with nongenetic environmentally interactive factors or "triggers" (Jacobson, 1997). For example, a child might have a genetic predisposition for a particular trait (e.g., hearing loss) and an environmental event (e.g., a virus or lack of oxygen) might activate it. Because genetic transmission can be very complicated, a genetic counselor should be consulted if the family requires information about endogenous hearing impairments. Approximately 50% of congenital hearing impairments have no identifiable cause; it is speculated that about 90% of hearing impairments with no known cause are genetic in origin (Fritsch & Sommer, 1991).

Pappas (1998) has identified a condition called "delayed hereditary sensorineural hearing impairment." Children with this condition are born with normal hearing but develop a hearing impairment during the first 12 months of life; hearing may continue to decrease until about 6 years of age. Thus, parents may be reporting events accurately when they say, "my baby really seemed to hear and even said some words, and then he stopped responding to my voice and stopped talking." Because the child had some early and critical listening (data input) opportunities, he or she typically responds very well to auditory-based intervention even though the hearing impairment ultimately may become profound in degree. More than one child in a family may have delayed hereditary sensorineural hearing impairment; it appears to be recessive in nature (Pappas, 1998).

The second general classification for cause of hearing impairment is *exogenous* which means that the hearing impairment was caused by an external, not a genetic, event. Exogenous hearing impairments cannot be transmitted to offspring because they are caused by environmental events, not by the parents' genes. Examples of agents that cause exogenous hearing impairments include lack of oxygen, bacterial or viral infections, noise exposure, and medications that damage the inner ear.

Severity or Degree of Hearing Impairments

In addition to being classified by cause and time of onset, hearing impairments also can be categorized by severity, i.e., how much the hearing impairment blocks an infant's sound reception (Northern & Downs, 1991). Children with normal hearing sensitivity are able to distinguish sound intensities of 15 dB HL or less in a quiet room.

Distinguishing Audiometric (Degree) and Functional Definitions for Hard of Hearing and Deaf

The terms hard of hearing and deaf can be used in several ways. The most common use refers to degree of hearing loss as noted on an audiogram. From an *audiometric perspective*, a child is said to be hard of hearing if their thresholds are better than 70 dB HL, allowing some access to loud conversational speech without wearing hearing aids. A child is described as being audiometrically deaf if thresholds are worse than 70 dB HL on the audiogram, because conversational speech is not available at all without some form of amplification technology.

Another way to define the terms hard of hearing and deaf is to use a *functional perspective* as proposed by Mark Ross (Ross, Brackett, & Maxon, 1991). A child is defined as being functionally hard of hearing if their primary mode of learning language is auditory and their reception of environmental information is primarily auditory, independent of the degree of hearing loss or its time of onset. Hence, a child could have been born with a profound hearing loss, but if amplification technology and auditory-verbal intervention enabled him or her to learn language primarily through audition, then that child would be functionally hard of hearing.

A person is defined as functionally deaf if his or her primary mode for learning language and receiving environmental information is visual. Visual input includes lip reading, cued speech, and manual communication or sign language. Note that traditional oral programs can be as visually-based in their assumptions and teaching as manual communication programs. Many early intervention programs erroneously assume that children with hearing impairments cannot use amplified auditory input as their *primary* mode for learning.

Ross (Ross et al., 1991) further elaborates on his proposed functional definitions by stating that a child—or anyone—who is functionally hard of hearing is much more like a person with typical hearing, relative to how information is learned, than someone who is functionally deaf. People who are functionally hard of hearing access the auditory centers of the brain like those with typical hearing, but those who are functionally deaf do not. Ross further states that the quality and integrity of the audiologic management that a child receives from the beginning are the most important factors determining whether the child will be functionally hard of hearing or functionally deaf.

Audiometric definitions need not determine functional outcome! As we move into the next century and have greater access to the auditory centers of the brain through early identification, sophisticated amplification technology, and auditory-based teaching, it should be possible to ensure that children with all degrees of hearing loss are functionally hard of hearing.

The term hearing impairment is used in this book to describe any type and degree of hearing loss, regardless of its time of onset, degree, or function. Following is a discussion of severity of hearing loss.

Normal Hearing Sensitivity: 0 to +15 dB HL for Children

An adult is considered to have normal hearing sensitivity if his or her hearing threshold, or the level at which sound is first detected, is no poorer than 25 dB HL. A child, however, needs better hearing sensitivity than an adult to hear and develop the crucial word-sound distinctions of language. **To be able to detect the complete speech signal even at soft conversational levels, a child's hearing sensitivity must be 15 dB HL or better at all frequencies in both ears** (Dobie & Berlin, 1978).

Note that good hearing sensitivity does not guarantee good ability to discriminate or understand speech in the presence of background noise. **A child may appear to hear well in a soundproof audiologic test room or a quiet one-to-one communicative situation, but not hear equally well in a relatively noisy home or school setting.**

Minimal or Slight Hearing Impairment: 16 to 25 dB HL for Children

A child with a minimal, borderline, or slight hearing impairment may experience problems in the following areas (Northern & Downs, 1991):

1.   hearing faint or distant speech (in fact, at least 10% of classroom instruction may be missed);
2.   detecting subtle conversational cues that could cause the child to respond inappropriately;
3.   keeping up with fast-paced communicative interactions; and
4.   hearing the word-sound distinctions that comprise morphological markers for tense, plurality, possessives, and so on.

In addition, the child may appear immature and be more fatigued than peers due to the increased level of effort needed to hear (Anderson, 1991; Brackett, 1997; Pillai, 1997). Thus, a minimal hearing impairment may have *major* negative consequences for a child who needs to be able to hear a clear and complete speech signal to have access to spoken information. Unfortunately, many slight hearing impairments are not even identified due to less than favorable hearing screening environments and lack of information about the hearing sensitivity a child needs to learn language and to acquire knowledge.

Unilateral Hearing Impairment

A unilateral hearing impairment occurs when a person has one ear that has normal hearing sensitivity and the other ear has at least a mild permanent hearing impairment. Contrary to popular opinion that one ear is all that is necessary, a unilateral hearing impairment can pose significant problems. Over 50% of children with unilateral hearing impairments experience educational difficulties (Bess, Klee, & Culbertson, 1986). Auditory skills that are important for classroom listening, such as identifying speech in noise and localizing sound sources, are difficult for the unilateral listener. Even when speech is directed to the good ear, the child with a unilateral hearing loss has more difficulty understanding the message than does a child with two normal ears (Gravel, Kurtzberg, Stapells, Vaughan, & Wallace, 1989). The same difficulties that apply to the child with a slight hearing impairment, mentioned previously, apply to the child with a unilateral hearing impairment.

Differences in behavioral patterns between children with normal hearing and children with unilateral hearing impairment have been noted (Culbertson & Gilbert, 1986; Oyler, Oyler & Matkin, 1988; Stein, 1983). Children with unilateral hearing impairments have been described as being more distractible, more frustrated, more dependent, less attentive, and appearing less confident in the classroom than their peers with normal hearing. Behavior difficulties may be more obvious than hearing difficulties in the child who has a unilateral hearing impairment (Cargill & Flexer, 1991). Unfortunately, negative behavior patterns rarely are linked to hearing impairment because the child has one perfectly good ear, and thus is believed to be able to hear when he or she wants to. Moreover, a unilateral hearing loss may go undetected. It is important to note that the child with a unilateral hearing impairment who also experiences repeated ear infections is at extreme risk for educational and behavioral difficulties that result from unmanaged hearing impairment (Cargill & Flexer, 1991).

Mild Hearing Impairment: 26 to 40 dB HL

Without audiologic management, a child who experiences a 30 dB hearing impairment can miss 25 to 40% of the speech signal depending on the noise level in the environment, distance from the speaker, and the configuration of the hearing impairment (Mueller & Killion, 1990; Olsen, Hawkins, & Van Tassell, 1987). In addition, the child likely will not benefit from passive learning because he or she will be unable to overhear conversations.

Without the use of hearing technology, the child who has a 35 to 40 dB hearing impairment can miss up to 50% of class discussions, especially when voices are soft or far away. The child may develop a negative self-concept when he or she is repeatedly accused of "daydreaming," or "hearing when he or she wants to," or "not trying" (Ross, Brackett, & Maxon, 1991). The child may be more fatigued or irritable than peers due to the level of effort needed to listen during the day (Brackett, 1997).

Clearly, the label "mild" used to describe this degree of hearing impairment is misleading. Mild is not mild relative to the potentially devastating impact of not hearing clear speech. A child with an unmanaged mild hearing impairment is likely to be at least one grade level behind his or her peers (Matkin, 1981; Northern & Downs, 1991). What could an undetected and untreated mild hearing impairment do to a child who has multiple sensory deficits?

Moderate Hearing Impairment: 41 to 55 dB HL

Prior to effective hearing management, a child with a moderate hearing impairment might understand face-to-face conversational speech at a distance of 3 to 5 feet if content/topic and vocabulary are known; 50 to 75% of the speech signal can be missed with a 40 to 45 dB hearing impairment, and 80 to 100% might be missed with a 50 dB hearing impairment (Mueller & Killion, 1990). The child is likely to have a limited vocabulary, delayed or defective syntax, and imperfect speech production. Communication, maturity, and social interaction are likely to be negatively affected as well. Children with moderate hearing impairments who have not received appropriate early (and often continuing) intervention are likely to be at least two grade levels behind by fourth grade (Ross, Brackett, & Maxon, 1991).

Moderately Severe Hearing Impairment: 56 to 70 dB HL

If amplification technologies are not used, spoken communication must be very loud and very close to be minimally understood; a child with a 55 dB hearing impairment can miss 100% of classroom information (Matkin, 1981). If the child does not receive appropriate early and continuing intervention, he or she is likely to have marked difficulty in school and evidence significantly delayed language, syntax, reduced speech intelligibility, and perhaps an atonal voice quality. Social behaviors also are likely to be problematic.

Severe Hearing Impairment: 71 to 90 dB HL

Even though a child with a severe hearing impairment cannot hear conversational speech at all without amplification, with appropriately fitted amplification, that child should be able to detect **all** speech sounds as well as environmental sounds (Ling, 1989). Without appropriate early intervention (and early intervention includes the use of amplification technology—hearing aids and assistive listening devices—for children with any degree of hearing impairment), spoken language will not develop. With appropriate amplification and auditory-based intervention strategies, the child with a severe hearing impairment can be functionally hard of hearing and not functionally deaf and thus be able to learn and live in a mainstreamed environment, perhaps with the assistance of some support services (Brackett, 1997; Davis, 1990; Ling, 1989; Ross, Brackett, & Maxon, 1991).

Profound Hearing Impairment: 91 dB HL or greater

A person with a profound hearing impairment cannot hear sounds without amplification. However, very few people have absolutely no residual hearing. The vast majority of persons with profound hearing impairments do have some residual or remaining hearing. The ability of a child with a profound hearing impairment to benefit from amplified sound is dependent on many factors, including the (Goldberg & Flexer, 1993; Ling, 1989; Pollack, 1985; Ross, 1990; Ross, Brackett & Maxon, 1991):

- Audiometric configuration of the residual or remaining hearing. How much hearing does the child actually have and at what frequencies?
- Child's age when amplification was first fitted. The earlier a hearing impairment is identified and amplification fitted, the more likely the child will benefit from early auditory-based intervention.
- Appropriateness of hearing aid power, frequency range, and use of volume. Because a child is wearing hearing aids does not mean that they are fitted optimally to the child's hearing loss.
- Type and intensity of early intervention employed. The more that hearing, listening, and spoken language are emphasized, the better opportunity the child has to develop those skills for communication in a mainstreamed setting.
- Expectations and belief, by parents and professionals, in the child's capacity to develop auditory skills and spoken communication.

- Support system available to the child. Does the family choose to and is the family able to manage the hearing technologies, and to carry-over intervention strategies on a daily basis?
- An infant or child with a profound hearing loss should be referred for a cochlear implant evaluation; a cochlear implant could provide much better sound access to the brain than hearing aids.

These are crucial factors that allow some children with profound congenital hearing impairments to live and learn as functionally hard-of-hearing people in fully mainstreamed settings, while other children with profound hearing impairments have limited or no auditory and spoken language skills. *The degree of hearing impairment, alone, does not determine communicative function.*

Professionals who provide early intervention services need to be aware of the tendency to underestimate the negative impact of a minimal hearing impairment. Professionals also need to avoid unnecessarily ruling-out the tremendous advantages of accessing residual hearing when a child has a profound hearing impairment.

All degrees of hearing impairment must be clearly identified, their impact recognized, and hearing management initiated very quickly to minimize the potentially devastating consequences of the acoustic filter effect of hearing impairment. Later chapters in this book discuss the hearing aids, assistive listening technologies, cochlear implants, and listening strategies necessary to facilitate auditory function.

No hearing impairment is too slight not to warrant hearing management, and no hearing impairment is too great to neglect the value of accessing residual hearing.

■ SYNDROMES

A *syndrome* can be defined as a set of symptoms that together characterize a disease or disorder. Some syndromes have an associated hearing impairment. The reader is referred to Fritsch and Sommer (1991), Jacobson (1997), Northern and Downs (1991), and Pappas (1998) for a detailed listing and discussion of syndromes that often include hearing impairment.

The presence of one structural abnormality increases the probability of additional abnormalities. For example, pigmentation abnormalities, such as a white forelock or eyes of different colors, may accompany sensorineural hearing impairments (Waardenburg's syndrome). Skeletal abnormalities may signal the presence of a congenital conductive hearing impairment due to middle ear malformation. Significant visual deficits may occur with sensorineural hearing impairment.

Any time a child demonstrates a structural abnormality, hearing impairment should be ruled out as a co-existing factor. Conversely, any time hearing impairment is diagnosed in a child, vigilance should be maintained for additional anomalies.

Fritsch and Sommer (1991) reported that the most common additional disorders that children with hearing impairment experience include asthma, vision disturbance, neuropsychiatric problems, arthritis, heart trouble, mental retardation, cerebral palsy, and cleft palate.

Four major dominantly transmitted syndromes are:

1. *Treacher-Collins syndrome.* Primary diagnostic features include facial bone abnormalities such as depressed cheekbones, deformed pinna, receding chin, and large fishlike mouth with frequent dental abnormalities. Atresia (absence or closure) of the ear canal, malformation of the middle ear ossicles, and cleft palate are common. Not all features are present in persons with Treacher-Collins syndrome nor are all features equal in severity. Hearing impairment is primarily conductive but may include a sensorineural component.

2. *Crouzon's syndrome.* Major diagnostic features associated with Crouzon's syndrome include an abnormally shaped head characterized by a central prominence in the frontal region and a nose resembling a beak. The shape of the skull is determined by the premature closing of the cranial sutures. Pinna may be low-set, and structural abnormalities of the middle ear occur in about one third of the cases, causing conductive hearing impairment.

3. *Waardenburg's syndrome.* Major diagnostic features include a white forelock, lateral displacement of

medial canthi, prominence of the root of the nose, and occasionally cleft palate. Congenital sensorineural hearing impairment ranging from mild to profound is present in 50% of the children and may be unilateral, bilateral, and/or progressive.

4. *Alport's syndrome.* Alport's syndrome is a renal (kidney) disorder associated with hearing and vision problems. Males tend to be more severely affected than females, and the accompanying sensorineural hearing impairment is usually bilateral, high frequency, ranges from mild to severe, and occurs in 40–60% of the cases. Age of onset of the hearing impairment typically is in preadolescence.

The three most common recessively transmitted syndromes are:

1. *Usher's syndrome.* Usher's syndrome is the major syndrome that involves both hearing and vision disorders. There is a progressive impairment of vision beginning in the early teens or twenties with resultant narrowing of the visual field leading to eventual blindness. The hearing impairment is sensorineural, bilateral, moderate to severe in degree, and may vary in age of onset, severity, and speed of progression.

2. *Pendred's syndrome.* Pendred's syndrome is an endocrine-metabolic disorder that includes goiter (an enlarged thyroid gland) and moderate-to-profound hearing impairment that is usually detected in the first 2 years of life.

3. *Jervell and Lange-Nielsen syndrome.* This syndrome, also identified as Long Q-T syndrome (LQTS), displays a cardiovascular disorder accompanying severe-to-profound, symmetrical, congenital hearing impairment. The child may experience fainting attacks or seizures. During an attack no blood is expelled from the heart. Except for two abnormalities in electrocardiogram readings, the health of the child appears normal. Jervell's syndrome often has been diagnosed erroneously as a seizure disorder and thus treated improperly. Rather than being rare, Jervell's syndrome more often goes undiagnosed. If not treated, death can result. Therefore, if a child who has a profound, congenital sensorineural hearing impairment

also has fainting spells or seizures, an electrocardiogram (heart function analysis) should be performed.

Syndromes may have a *variable expression* which means that the number and severity of the symptoms vary from person to person.

■ AUDITORY PATHOLOGIES

Conductive Hearing Impairments

In conductive hearing impairments, the location of the damage that causes the hearing impairment (also called the site of lesion) occurs in the outer and/or middle ear. Because the conductive mechanism functions to conduct or transmit sound to the inner ear and does not contain irreplaceable nerve endings, many conductive pathologies can be treated by medical or surgical intervention.

Conductive hearing impairments typically involve both medical and educational issues. The medical issue is relevant because the infant or child may have a pathology that affects general health. Furthermore, medical treatment often can restore the hearing that has been impaired by a disease located in the outer or middle ear. The educational component also is crucial because the conductive hearing loss can have an impact on language acquisition and educational performance.

The conductive hearing losses most common to infants and toddlers include: otitis media, collapsed ear canals, abnormalities of the middle ear ossicles, atresia, stenosis, cerumen impaction, otitis externa, perforated tympanic membrane, objects in the ear canal, cholesteatoma, and mastoiditis.

Otitis Media (Commonly Called Middle Ear Infection)

Ear infections are the most common cause of conductive hearing loss and hearing problems in children. *In fact, infants and children with otitis media are the largest population who can benefit from the listening strategies detailed in this book.*

Otitis media is an inflammation of the middle ear. Otitis media with effusion (OME) is an inflammation of the middle ear that includes fluid in the normally air-filled middle ear space (Paradise, 1980). This fluid may occur with or without active infection, but it almost always causes hearing problems. Acute otitis media (AOM) is a middle ear infection of recent onset, accompanied by symptoms and signs of infection (fever, pain, irritability), and lasting 2 to 3 weeks. Subacute otitis media is an ear infection that fails to clear and lasts for 3 weeks to 3 months, usually with effusion. Chronic otitis media is otitis media of more than 3 months duration with or without tympanic membrane perforation (hole in the eardrum) and drainage.

About one half of the episodes of OME are "silent" and undetected by a parent because the child does not appear to be sick. Fluid, which causes hearing problems, is present in the middle ear but there is no infection in the fluid. Hence, when a baby is brought to the pediatrician for a well-baby visit, OME is surprisingly discovered almost 50% of the time (Friel-Patti, Finitzo, Formby, & Brown, 1987; Gravel, Wallace, & Abraham, 1991). These unrecognized bouts of OME mean that parents are not necessarily accurate reporters of their child's history of middle ear dysfunction.

Otitis media is a major public health problem in the United States with almost 4 billion dollars per year spent in treatment and research; about 2 billion dollars per year is spent on surgical intervention. Estimated direct and indirect management costs are about $406 per patient episode, with cost of myringotomy with insertion of tympanostomy tubes $2,174 (U.S. Department of Health and Human Services, 1994). Otitis media is the most common reason for children's visits to physicians other than for checkups (Bluestone et al., 1983). Between 1975 and 1990, office visits for otitis media increased by 150% (to 24.5 million), with children under 15 years of age accounting for 81% of the visits. Children under 2 years of age had the highest rate of visits to physician offices for otitis media, with a 224% increase from 1975 to 1990 (U.S. Department of Health and Human Services, 1994). At least 75% of the children seen by pediatricians have had at least one episode of OME by age two, with age two and under comprising the major at-risk population (Baker, 1991; Garrard & Clark, 1985). The incidence increases to 85% of all school-age children having had at least one episode. By age three, 33% of the population has had three or more bouts of OME (Bluestone et al., 1983). Unfortunately, the younger a child is when the first bout occurs, the greater the likelihood of recurrent and severe episodes (Gravel et al., 1989; Warren & Stool, 1971). The reason is that the disease process of OME actually alters the structure of the middle ear lining (Tos, Holm-Jensen, Sorensen, & Morgensen, 1982), with recovery occurring more slowly with younger age and with each additional ear infection.

CAUSES AND EFFECTS OF EAR INFECTIONS. A malfunctioning Eustachian tube is the cause of OME, with viral upper respiratory infections being the typical precursors of that malfunction. The usual pattern is for an ear infection to occur a few days after the onset of a cold or other upper respiratory infection. The infection causes mucus to obstruct the function of the Eustachian tube.

The Eustachian tube, a tiny structure (1 cm long) that connects the back of the throat with the middle ear, is comprised of cartilage and muscle and includes a flutter valve opening. The Eustachian tube has three main functions: equalizing air pressure differences between the middle ear and the environment, protecting the delicate middle ear from secretions from the nose and throat, and draining the normal secretions from the middle ear cavity into the throat (Paradise, 1980; Stach, 1998). Pressure regulation is its most important function. If the Eustachian tube fails, normal atmospheric pressure is not maintained in the middle ear, negative pressure then develops which often leads to fluid build-up due to the near vacuum "sucking" fluid out of the mucous lining of the middle ear cavity. Fluid can exist "silently," causing decreased hearing, or it can become infected with bacteria and/or viruses. These in turn cause illness (fever, pain) and hearing impairment.

To reiterate, a conductive hearing loss typically accompanies ear infections. Hearing impairment can occur even when fluid is not present but high negative pressure exists in the middle ear (Bluestone et al., 1983). The average hearing impairment is 25 dB, but it can increase to 50 dB (Paradise, 1981). The hearing loss may be more severe at some frequencies than others. Fluid and/or negative pressure in the middle ear, both with coexisting hearing impairment, may persist from 2 weeks to 3 months following a single bout of OME (Northern & Downs, 1991; Teele, 1991). If a child is otitis-prone (has recurring ear infections), the child may have constant middle ear fluid. Therefore, some children with OME may have temporary, fluctuating hearing impairment, while others have long-term hearing losses (Hayes & Northern, 1996; Sheehy, 1983).

HIGH INCIDENCE POPULATIONS. Harrison and Belhorn (1991) summarized conditions and situations that predispose a child to become otitis prone:

1. Congenital abnormalities. Cleft palate *(even after repair)*, congenital cytomegalovirus (CMV), perinatally acquired HIV infection, and other immune deficiencies.

2. Genetic factors such as Down syndrome.
3. Specific infections, especially upper respiratory infections—incompletely treated sinusitis and purulent conjunctivitis. Both bacteria and viruses seem to be involved.
4. Historical factors. First bout of otitis media with effusion occurs before 6 months of age and more than three episodes of otitis media with effusion in the previous 6 months.
5. Environmental factors. Attendance at a day-care center and passive smoking.

OME can be quite complex. Allergies are a factor in 30 to 40% of cases of recurrent OME. Some children have an immune deficiency that does not allow their body to fight the resultant bacterial or viral infection.

Some populations have a high incidence of associated OME (Downs, 1980). Children who were in neonatal intensive care units (NICUs) as infants have an incidence of approximately 80% (Berman, Balkany, & Simmons, 1978). Infants often are in NICUs due to respiratory difficulties with resultant naso-tracheal intubation (i.e., a small tube is inserted through the infant's nose into the trachea to assist in breathing). The tube often occludes the opening of the Eustachian tube at the back of the throat behind the nose. The presence of the tube for a period of time can cause Eustachian tube malfunction with resultant OME. Thus, an infant who has been in an NICU for several weeks might leave the hospital with OME and hearing impairment. Because the younger the child is when the first bout occurs, the greater the likelihood of recurrent episodes, children with NICU backgrounds can become otitis-prone (Gravel, McCarton, & Ruben, 1988). Thus, a cycle is set in motion with a child having continual ear infections, continual middle ear fluid, and *continual hearing impairment.*

Many infants and young children who qualify for early intervention programming are graduates of NICUs; they are therefore at risk for recurrent OME. Remember, OME is a medical *and* an educational problem, with a child's health and language development both at risk. Neither issue can be ignored, nor can treatment of one substitute for treatment of the other (Downs, Jafek, & Wood, 1981).

Another population with a high incidence of OME includes children with cleft palate, who have almost a 100% probability of

OME while the cleft is unrepaired (Paradise & Bluestone, 1974; Pappas, 1998). The reason for this very high incidence is that the same muscles that control the flutter valve opening of the Eustachian tube are connected to the soft palate. Children with cleft palate typically are plagued with OME with resultant hearing impairment throughout childhood.

Children with Down syndrome have at least an 88% incidence rate of OME and other conductive pathologies (Dahle & McCollister, 1986; Kaga & Marsh, 1986; Maurizi, Ottaviani, Paludetti, & Lungarotti, 1985; Strome, 1981). Structurally, the position of the Eustachian tube often appears abnormal as does the actual middle ear space and associated ossicles (Balkany, Mischke, Downs, & Jafek, 1979; Harada & Sando, 1981). In addition, the ear canals are often stenotic (abnormally small), causing even a small amount of cerumen (ear wax) to totally block the opening. The high incidence of upper respiratory infections also contributes to high incidence of OME.

A child with Down syndrome has a high likelihood of having an essentially permanent conductive hearing impairment. Three out of four children with Down syndrome in an early intervention program probably have hearing impairments which, if unmanaged, present a major barrier to the language-learning process.

One in four children with learning disabilities, twice the number in the non-learning-disabled population, have recurrent OME (Reichman & Healy, 1983). This figure is not surprising due to the subtle negative effects of word-sound confusions caused by even a mild hearing impairment. If a child cannot hear the unstressed linguistic markers that denote plurality, tense, or verb changes, it will be difficult for him or her to learn these concepts.

The presence of hearing impairment during the first year of life is associated with attention and language-learning problems even if hearing loss is temporary (Northern & Downs, 1991). Gravel, Wallace, and Abraham (1991) found that children with early hearing impairment caused by OME may not develop a strong auditory base and cannot tolerate low levels of acoustic or linguistic redundancy. Nozza, Rossman, Bond, and Miller (1990) reported that children who experienced OME during their first year may have difficulty learning to distinguish individual phonemes because the presence of even a slight hearing impairment necessitates a more favorable speech-to-noise ratio than is available in typical communication environments. Cranford, Thompson, Hoyer, and Faires (1997) found that older children with severe histories of OME before the age of three were impaired in their ability to discriminate the frequency of short duration tones—an analytic function that is critical for normal speech understanding. These findings highlight the fact that early otitis media could have long-term negative effects.

MEDICAL DIAGNOSIS AND TREATMENT OF OME. Medical diagnosis of ear infections is most reliably made through the use of pneumatic otoscopy; an otoscope with a bulb and tube attached is used to blow small puffs of air through the ear canal causing the eardrum to move (Baker, 1991; Berman, Balkany, & Simmons, 1978). Both visual inspection (color and shape) and mobility of the eardrum contribute to an accurate medical diagnosis. A fluid-filled middle ear will not allow the eardrum to move well, if at all. It should be remembered that infant eardrums often are very difficult to visualize due to their horizontal position when compared to adult eardrums (Johnson, 1961; McLellan & Webb, 1961; Wright, 1997).

Physicians also rely on behavioral symptoms and other case history information (Baker, 1991; Snow, 1979). Children may manifest general symptoms such as irritability, listlessness, and distractibility or more specific "ear" symptoms such as pulling on the ears, head banging, and rolling the head from side to side. Of these symptoms, irritability is the most common.

Medical management of OME is complex. Routine nonsurgical intervention consists of antibiotics such as Amoxicillin™, Trimethoprim-sulfamethoxazole (such as Bactrim™ or Septra™), Ceftin™, Cefzil™, Augmentin™, Ceclor™, Suprax™, and Pediazole™ (Baker, 1991; Garrard & Clark, 1985; Pashley, 1984). Amoxicillin™ continues to be the most common and least expensive antibiotic prescribed. All of these antibiotics only sterilize the middle ear fluid of bacteria; they do not necessarily eliminate the fluid. Interestingly, antihistamines and decongestants have been shown to be of limited or no value in treating OME (Pashley, 1984).

Antibiotics, particularly Amoxicillin™, can be used in a preventative fashion for some children who are prone to having ear infections (Cotton, 1991; Pappas, 1998; Teele, 1991). The child can be given a daily dose during the winter months to try to prevent ear infections from occurring. In addition, an influenza vaccination may prevent otitis media that results from the influenza virus. Steroids, such as prednisone, have been used successfully for a short period of time (6–10 days) along with antibiotics to help reduce the inflammation caused by ear infections in some children.

A federal panel of health care experts issued guidelines for otitis media, recommending that physicians should opt for a period of "watchful waiting" rather than administering medications or doing surgery when dealing with most cases of noninfectious otitis media among otherwise healthy 1- to 3-year-olds (U.S. Department of Health and Human Services, 1994). The panel was influenced by data suggesting that noninfectious otitis media usually clears up by itself in 3 to 6 months. These guidelines recommend hearing tests and antibiotics only if the symptoms of otitis media persist after 3 months, and surgery to insert PE tubes if symptoms are present for more than 6 months. Note that these guidelines apply only to otitis media with effusion, and not to acute otitis media. "Watchful waiting" also does *not* apply to children who have sensorineural hearing loss, developmental delay, craniofacial anomalies, language problems, and other health issues; such children require more vigorous medical management. Surgical intervention typically is recommended if the young child has had (a) three or more medically diagnosed bouts of otitis media within a 6-month interval; (b) structural changes in the tympanic membrane, such as a retraction pocket or atrophy; (c) chronic otitis media with history of more than one perforation; and (d) concurrent sensorineural hearing loss and persistent negative middle-ear pressure (Pappas, 1998).

The surgery, called tympanostomy, consists of making an incision through the eardrum, suctioning the fluid out of the middle ear, and then inserting tympanostomy tubes (also called ventilating tubes or PE tubes) through the tympanic membrane (Cotton, 1991). These tubes substitute for the malfunctioning Eustachian tubes, providing air to the middle ear space (see Figure 3–2).

The insertion of ventilating tubes is the most popular surgical procedure performed in the United States under a general anesthetic; there are approximately 1 million surgeries per year and over 50 different styles of ventilating tubes (Cotton, 1991; Teele, 1991). The surgery takes about 10 minutes and is regarded as a very safe procedure. The procedure does require a general anesthetic and could result in some scarring of the eardrum with repeated tube insertions (Bluestone et al., 1983; Cotton, 1991; Draf & Schulz, 1980; Paradise, 1981). In addition, the tubes must be carefully managed by keeping the ear canals clean and dry to avoid further infection. Tympanostomy tubes typically fall out naturally from 6 to 18 months after insertion. They may need to be surgically replaced if infections continue.

Persistent OME can have complications such as cholesteatoma (nonmalignant middle ear tumor), meningitis, and perma-

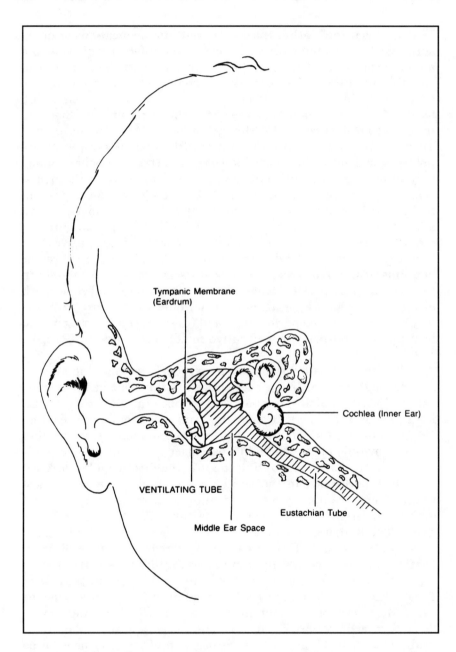

Labels within the figure:

Tympanic Membrane (Eardrum)

Cochlea (Inner Ear)

VENTILATING TUBE

Eustachian Tube

Middle Ear Space

Figure 3–2. Tympanostomy (ventilating) tubes, surgically inserted through the eardrum, replace malfunctioning Eustachian tube, allowing ventilation of the middle ear space. (Illustration by Jackie Rios)

nent hearing impairment resulting from the toxins seeping into the delicate inner ear (Northern, 1996; Ruben & Math, 1978). Appropriate medical management needs to be carefully evaluated for each individual child. There is no simple answer.

AUDIOLOGIC DIAGNOSIS AND TREATMENT OF OTITIS MEDIA. The two main purposes of pediatric audiologic evaluation are: (a) the evaluation of hearing sensitivity and (b) the evaluation of auditory behaviors (i.e., does the child respond to sound as one would expect of an infant or child of this particular developmental age?) (Jerger, 1984; Martin & Clark, 1996; Northern & Downs, 1991).

The diagnosis of middle ear disease is a medical and not an audiologic prerogative. Therefore, the audiologic diagnosis of the hearing impairment caused by otitis media does not differ from the diagnosis of hearing impairment caused by any other pathology. Treatment of the hearing impairment, not treatment of disease, is the purview of the audiologist.

Physicians are trained to deal with the medical and surgical diagnosis and management of hearing impairment. Audiologists address the habilitative issues of hearing impairment: What is the type and degree of hearing impairment? How does the hearing impairment affect the child's life? What audiologic strategies can be employed to mitigate the effects of the hearing impairment?

The specific hearing tests employed in a pediatric test battery will be discussed in Chapter 4. At this point, suffice it to say that a test battery approach, using multiple behavioral and objective tests based on a child's developmental not chronological age, is crucial (Jerger, 1984; Martin & Clark, 1996; Stach, 1998). Typically, more than one test session is needed to obtain accurate data about the child's hearing impairment.

The audiologic/educational intervention for the hearing impairment caused by ear infections typically does not vary from interventions employed for other hearing impairments, because it is the hearing impairment, not the disease, that is at issue. Audiologic interventions are used in addition to, not instead of, medical interventions. Audiologic interventions, which are detailed in Chapters 5, 6, and 7, include amplification (hearing aids and assistive listening devices), speaking very close to or directly into the ear of the child, increasing the melody or prosodic changes in the parents' and clinicians' voices, incorporating auditory/listening skills into daily activities, increasing language stimulation, and parent education and training.

Although the effects of continuing, persistent, and current hearing impairment are more definite (Paden, Novak, & Beiter, 1987), the negative effects of early and fluctuating hearing impairment are influenced by many factors (Friel-Patti et al., 1987; Paradise, 1981; Ventry, 1980). Individual child differences are the product of a constellation of other variables acting in tandem with hearing impairment. These factors include irregular medical management, low socioeconomic level, large family size, general malaise caused by illness, effectiveness of the child's cognitive style, and reduced parental linguistic interaction due to nonresponsiveness of the child (Silva, Chalmers, & Stewart, 1986). These additional factors make it difficult to predict accurately in advance how devastating a fluctuating hearing impairment will be on a particular child's later verbal and academic performance. Nevertheless, Gravel and Wallace (1992) found that children with positive histories of otitis media during their first year of life required a more advantageous S/N ratio to perform at 50% sentence intelligibility than did their otitis negative peers. It therefore seems prudent to initiate early intervention routinely for hearing impairment, in an attempt to prevent later difficulties, rather than wait to see whether difficulties develop and then try to remediate them.

Following is a discussion of other conductive hearing losses in children.

Collapsed Ear Canals

Many infants and young children have very soft and small ear canals that can close or collapse as a result of the pressure caused by earphones applied during hearing tests. The result of ear canal collapse is an erroneous conductive hearing impairment. Audiometric results indicate a conductive hearing loss that does not really exist. The suspected hearing loss will not be confirmed by case history, immittance audiometry (an objective test), or medical examination of the ear. Such children can be shown to have normal hearing when tested in a sound field (the sound is transmitted into the test room through loudspeakers without using earphones), or with hand-held earphones (to avoid earphone pressure on the ear canal). The most effective way to measure the hearing in each ear and to avoid collapsing ear canals is to use insert earphones and not the typical earphones that fit over the ears (Stach, 1998). Earphone types will be discussed and pictured in Chapter 4.

Ossicular Abnormalities

Ossicular abnormalities are a type of birth defect that did not allow for the precise formation of the tiny middle ear bones. Surgery can correct the problem in some cases, but is typically not elected for children due to the danger of cutting the facial nerve. Damaging the facial nerve can cause facial paralysis. Therefore, hearing aids often are the preferred treatment. Hearing aids can be very effective for a conductive hearing impairment because amplification essentially must overcome only the conductive barrier without having to deal with the distortion caused by a sensory impairment.

Atresia

Causing a complete closure of the ear canal, atresia is a type of birth defect. Clearly, if the ear canal is absent or blocked, sound cannot be conducted to the middle and inner ear. Because of the unknown position of the facial nerve in cases of atresia, surgery often is not recommended because facial paralysis could result. Amplification typically is recommended. Atresia typically is unilateral (occurring on one side). Audiological management for unilateral hearing impairment, such as using an FM system fitted to the good ear, should be employed (Cargill & Flexer, 1991).

Stenotic Ear Canal

A stenotic ear canal is one that is abnormally small and narrow. Small amounts of cerumen or ear wax can completely block the ear canal causing hearing loss. A child with stenosis may function as if he or she is wearing earplugs. Physical examination of the health of the eardrum also is very difficult as is the comfortable fitting of earmolds for hearing aids. What appears to be a trivial problem can be the source of constant discomfort and hearing loss.

Cerumen or Ear Wax Impaction

The production of ear wax is a normal process. Ear wax protects and cleanses the delicate ear canal. Ear wax varies in color and consistency and can look like blood clots, black tar, yellow crayon, white rocks, or amber liquid. New cerumen is typically gold in color, and "old" cerumen is very dark due to oxidation.

Normally, ear wax is moved by the cells lining the ear canal to the opening in the pinna where it typically dries and flakes away.

The use of Q-tips to remove wax is potentially dangerous because the wax is forced back into the ear canal, thereby interfering with the natural cleansing process.

Some individuals produce a great deal of wax which can block the ear canal. This wax needs to be removed, typically by a physician although the Audiology scope of practice has expanded to include routine cerumen removal (AAA, 1997; Roeser & Crandell, 1991). Because cerumen glands are similar to sweat glands, emotional states and medications, as well as genetic makeup, can influence the amount of secretion.

The hearing loss caused by partial cerumen impaction (a lot of ear wax but the ear canal is not blocked totally) is high frequency in nature. Complete cerumen impaction or blockage results in a 30 to 50 dB HL hearing impairment across all frequencies (Roeser & Crandell, 1991). Approximately 10% of children and about 30% of persons with developmental disabilities have cerumen problems that cause hearing loss until the cerumen is removed (Crandell & Roeser, 1993). Impacted cerumen also can cause tinnitus (ringing in the ears), dizziness, itching, earache, otitis externa (infection in the ear canal), cardiac depression, and chronic cough.

The wearing of hearing aids (specifically earmolds) may interfere with the natural cleansing process in the ear canal because the presence of the earmold can push the wax back into the ear canal. For this reason, it is important to be aware that infants and toddlers who wear hearing aids need to be monitored for excess cerumen that can interfere with amplification by blocking the ear canal or by plugging up the earmold.

What appears to be a trivial problem, excessive ear wax, may cause hearing loss in as many as 30% of the infants and young children in early intervention programs. Any hearing impairment could sabotage the child's opportunity to develop spoken communication.

Otitis Externa

Otitis externa simply means an infection of the ear canal, such as swimmer's ear. If moisture collects in the ear canal, it can form the basis for a bacterial or fungal infection with resultant pain, swelling, and drainage. Medical treatment is necessary. Otitis externa is a problem for children who wear hearing aids because the earmold causes discomfort and interferes with healing. Amplification typically is discontinued to allow air into the ear canal until the infection is cleared, causing a valuable loss of educational time. Good ear hygiene must be observed by keeping the ear canals clean and dry and washing earmolds regularly in mild soapy detergent to minimize the spread of infection.

Perforated Tympanic Membrane

A tympanic perforation is a hole in the eardrum, most often caused by ear infection but also by trauma. A sharp blow to the ear may rupture the eardrum as well as damage the ossicles behind it. There also may be drainage from the middle ear through the perforation. The perforation may heal by itself or require surgical repair. It causes varying degrees of hearing loss depending on size and location (Pappas, 1998).

Objects in the Ear Canal

It is not unusual for a small child to push objects into the ear canal. Things such as hairpins, cereal, marbles, rocks, earrings, small hearing aid batteries, bugs, beads, and other food and toys have been removed from children's ear canals. These objects can cause discomfort, infection, and/or hearing loss. They typically are removed by a physician.

Cholesteatoma

A cholesteatoma is a nonmalignant tumor that may grow from a perforated eardrum. A child can be born with a cholesteatoma, but most often the tumor results from chronic ear infections. It must be surgically removed because it can become a threat to health and cause hearing impairment. The prevention of this tumor is one reason for diligent medical management of ear infections.

Mastoiditis

Mastoiditis is an infection of the mastoid process, which is the bony projection behind the pinna. Prior to the discovery of antibiotics, the spread of ear infections from the middle ear space to the mastoid was common. Mastoiditis often necessitated a mastoidectomy which is a surgical procedure that literally cleared out the entire middle ear space causing significant hearing impairment. Fortunately, good medical management of otitis media now helps avoid mastoiditis.

Sensorineural Hearing Impairments

A sensorineural hearing impairment is caused by pathology or damage that occurs in the inner ear or cochlea, which is the part of the ear housing thousands of tiny sensory receptors called hair cells. This damage is permanent; there is no medical treatment. Hearing aids or cochlear implants and assistive listening devices typically are recommended to help mitigate the effects of sensorineural hearing impairments. Amplification, however, cannot correct the damage to the inner ear. Rather, hearing aids amplify and shape incoming sounds to make them audible to an ear that cannot otherwise detect them.

Some of the more common causes of sensorineural hearing impairments in children are defined and detailed in the following sections. They include: noise-induced hearing impairment, viral and bacterial infections such as cytomegalovirus and meningitis, anoxia, ototoxicity, large vestibular aqueduct, perilymphatic fistula, and Rh incompatibility.

Tinnitus

Tinnitus often is associated with sensorineural hearing impairment. Tinnitus is hearing ringing, buzzing, roaring, or chirping sounds. Tinnitus can occur in children. Ringing can be constant or infrequent and can range from barely noticeable to terribly distracting. Not much is known about child behaviors that occur in response to tinnitus, but adults can be debilitated by its presence (White, Hoffman, & Gale, 1986).

Noise-Induced Hearing Impairment

Noise induced hearing impairment (permanent inner ear damage caused by prolonged exposure to loud sounds), although not prevalent in babies, has been linked to loud sounds occurring in incubators. Average noise levels in incubators have been reported to be greater than 60 dB, and opening and closing the unit doors can create peak amplitudes of 114 dB (Bess, Peek, & Chapman, 1979).

Unfortunately, hearing impairment due to exposure to loud sounds, such as music, has increased in young children. Chermak, Curtis, and Seikel (1996) reported that even young, primary-level children should be educated about the hazards of exposure to loud sounds and subsequently receive training about how to protect their ears.

Viral and Bacterial Infections

Some infections are transferred from a pregnant mother to her fetus through the placenta. The mother may or may not feel ill herself, and the negative effects on her fetus vary. Hearing impairment may range from mild to profound. Minimal to serious additional abnormalities may be present. Exposure to infection often is discovered through blood tests. Examples of in utero infections include cytomegalovirus, rubella, herpes, toxoplasmosis, and syphilis.

Children also may develop a hearing impairment from infections acquired after birth. Bacterial meningitis is the worst culprit because the hearing impairment may not be apparent until months after the child has left the hospital.

MENINGITIS. Meningitis, an inflammation of the coverings (meninges) of the brain and its fluids, is primarily a disease of the central nervous system. Bacterial meningitis has been the most common cause of acquired hearing loss in infancy and childhood (Pappas, 1998). Symptoms of meningitis include fever, headache, neck stiffness, irritability, altered consciousness, and vomiting. A lumbar puncture (spinal tap) is necessary to make a definite diagnosis. The hearing loss that results from meningitis is caused by inflammation of the membranous structures of the cochlea due to the extension of the infection from the meninges (Pappas, 1998). Over time the cochlea could ossify, causing complete hearing loss. Fortunately, a cochlear implant, if inserted before complete ossification of the cochlea (as shown in a CT scan), can allow hearing to be available to many children through direct simulation of auditory neural tissue (Estabrooks, 1998). Cochlear implants will be discussed in Chapter 5.

Hearing loss in postmeningitic children varies in amount, symmetry, and configuration; many patients demonstrate a fluctuating but progressive hearing loss (Pappas, 1998). Careful and ongoing audiologic monitoring and management are essential for all children who have had bacterial meningitis, especially *H. influenza* (ASHA, 1991c).

CYTOMEGALOVIRUS (CMV). Congenital CMV infection is believed to be the primary cause of viral-type congenital sensorineural hearing impairments in the United States (Johnson, Williamson, & Chmiel, 1991). Studies have projected that approximately 40,000 children with congenital CMV will be born each year, and about 15% of the infected infants, or 6,000 children, likely will experience sensorineural hearing impairment (Williamson et al.,

1990). Hearing impairment can be stable, fluctuating, progressive, bilateral or unilateral, and range in severity from mild to profound. Mild hearing losses are likely to be progressive in severity (Pappas, 1998). Consequently, the child with suspected CMV involvement requires consistent audiologic evaluations and flexible amplification fitting.

CMV is a member of the herpes virus family that also includes herpes simplex virus (cold sores), varicella-zoster virus (chickenpox and shingles), and Epstein Barr virus (mononucleosis); these viruses all have the ability to cause latent infections because they can persist in the body indefinitely (Kinney, Onorato, & Stewart, 1985). Therefore, the maternal infection that is transmitted to the fetus in a congenital infection could be either primary (first-time infection) or recurrent (reactivation of a previous infection). Neonates who are symptomatic at birth are probably born to mothers who experienced primary CMV infections during pregnancy. CMV is a very common virus infecting nearly all people at some time during their lifetimes without negative consequences.

Approximately 10% of infants with CMV are symptomatic at birth. Symptoms can include central nervous system disabilities, hearing impairment, visual disorders, developmental delay, psychomotor retardation, enlarged liver and spleen, decreased platelet count in the blood, inflammation of the retina, cerebral palsy, and language or learning disorders. In an infected person, CMV can be found in the saliva, urine, blood, tears, stool, cervical secretions, and semen; an infected person (with or without obvious symptoms) can secrete CMV for many months or years (Eichhorn, 1982). Note that many apparently healthy infants and children can be actively secreting CMV. Infection control procedures, which include regular handwashing, should be routinely employed when working in clinical/educational settings (ASHA, 1991b).

Anoxia

Anoxia is lack of oxygen, a condition that can occur before, during, or shortly after birth. Low birth weight (<1,500 grams) also can contribute to respiratory problems. There is a unique audiometric configuration suggestive of anoxia, which consists of essentially normal low-frequency (pitch) hearing, which sharply drops to a more severe hearing impairment in the higher frequencies. With this configuration, an infant or toddler "hears" sounds, but is

unable to distinguish individual speech sounds, especially consonants. High-frequency hearing loss is difficult to recognize because
a child seems to respond to sound. Hearing impairment often is
overlooked or prematurely ruled out (Coplan, 1987), because the
child evidences audibility but not intelligibility.

**Any child with a history of anoxia or low birth weight
needs repeated hearing tests with particular emphasis to
high-frequency hearing.**

Ototoxicity

Ototoxicity is a "poisoning" of the delicate inner ear by high doses
of some medications such as mycin drugs (e.g., kanamycin, gen-
tamicin, tobramycin, amikacin, and neomycin), some diuretics,
quinine, cisplatin (a chemotherapeutic agent effective in the treatment of cancer), and aspirin. Mycin drugs, taken in conjunction
with loop diuretics have proved particularly problematic (Northern, 1996). The term "high dose" is relative, because a normal dose
for a 130-pound woman would be abnormally high for a 1-pound
fetus. Thus, ototoxic drugs can be administered directly to a child,
usually as a life-saving measure, or can be transmitted to the fetus
in utero through medications taken by the mother.

Ototoxic hearing impairments most often are permanent, but
can be fluctuating such as those caused by aspirin. The hearing
impairment typically is high frequency, but may include mid-fre-
quencies. Most important, ototoxic hearing impairments may have
a *delayed onset*, so hearing sensitivity must be monitored even
after medication has been discontinued.

Large Vestibular Aqueduct

Large vestibular aqueduct is a congenital malformation of the temporal bone that predisposes the affected person to early onset
hearing loss; a vestibular aqueduct diameter larger than 1.5 mm
to 2.0 mm is generally considered to be the defining characteristic
as identified through a CT scan (Cox & McDonald, 1996).

Several theories have been proposed to explain the resultant
hearing loss. One theory suggests that the hearing loss results
from cerebrospinal fluid pressure fluctuations transmitted by the
endolymphatic duct to the scala media (of the cochlea/inner ear) or
through the lateral wall of the internal auditory canal. Another
theory proposes that a large vestibular aqueduct is a variation of a

Mondini dysplasia with a high incidence of round window abnormalities; these may predispose the patient to perilymph fistulas that could be the actual cause of the sensorineural hearing loss (Cox & MacDonald, 1996). Hearing loss may be unilateral or bilateral, variable, fluctuating, and with a tendency to progress to a profound level (Pappas, 1998). Events such as minor head trauma have been reported as possible triggers for decreases in hearing. A CT scan is necessary for a positive medical diagnosis. While it seems that large vestibular aqueduct is rare, the actual prevalence may be much higher than expected because CT scans are not performed routinely.

Audiologists should be aware that children or adolescents who have a sensorineural hearing loss of unknown cause, with or without accompanying dizziness, may have a large vestibular aqueduct, especially if their hearing loss is progressive (Cox & MacDonald, 1996). Theoretically, the onset or progression of the hearing loss could be delayed by changes in patient behavior at an early age to reduce bumps to the head (Pappas, 1998). Hearing must be monitored closely. If hearing loss progresses to the severe to profound range, a cochlear implant should be considered (Estabrooks, 1998).

Perilymphatic Fistula (PLF)

A perilymphatic fistula is a leak in the oval or round window. Both are points of communication between the middle and inner ear. Specifically, the leak causes the delicately balanced fluid in the inner ear to seep out, interrupting the function of the organ of Corti which is housed in the cochlea. PLF may be caused by a congenital weakness or defect in the bony partition between the perilymphatic compartment of the inner ear and the middle ear or it may be produced by a traumatic event such as a head injury or sudden barometric change. A fistula can cause a sudden and dramatic hearing impairment or an increase in the severity of an existing hearing loss. Diagnosis and surgical repair must be virtually immediate to preserve hearing. Although once thought to occur mostly in older adults, there is now evidence that fistulas are a problem for young children as well (Myer, Farrer, Drake, & Cotton, 1989; Pappas & Schneiderman, 1989).

An important issue to note is that definite diagnosis can be made only through surgical exploration of the middle ear. Many physicians are reluctant to perform an invasive procedure as a diagnostic tool because there is a high incidence of natural hearing impairment progression in children with sensorineural hearing impairment (Pappas, 1998). That is, fluctuating and/or progressive hearing impairments have been associated with genetic hearing impairment (both dominant and recessive), ototoxicity, meningitis, CMV, and meningitis as well as with PLF.

Pappas and Schneiderman (1989) reached the following conclusions about PLF:

1. Unless progression of a pre-existing sensorineural hearing impairment is accompanied by inner ear defects that have been documented by a CT scan, craniofacial abnormalities, progression of hearing impairment greater than 25 dB, disequilibrium, or history of antecedent trauma, surgery is not recommended.

2. Children with demonstrated inner ear defects should avoid activities such as contact sports, weightlifting, kayaking, scuba diving, and deep diving into a pool.

3. A PLF in one ear increases the chance of a PLF in the other ear.

4. When middle ear pathology coexists with permanent sensorineural hearing impairment, changing sensorineural hearing levels are often difficult to identify.

Acoustic Neuroma

Also called an VIIIth nerve tumor, an acoustic neuroma is a nonmalignant tumor that grows off of the main nerve trunk that carries auditory sensations from the inner ear to the brain. A neuroma can develop into a brainstem tumor that causes hearing impairment and could be fatal if not diagnosed and surgically removed.

Rh Incompatibility

Rh incompatibility involves the destruction of Rh positive blood cells of the fetus by maternal antibodies. Complications can include hearing impairment, jaundice, and possible brain damage. Fortunately, due to medical advances, Rh incompatibility like rubella is no longer a primary cause of sensorineural hearing impairment in children (Upfold, 1988).

Dysplasias

Dysplasias are malformations or incomplete development of the inner ear (cochlea). Many anatomic abnormalities of the inner ear are associated with hearing impairment. The three most common dysplasias include (Pappas, 1998):

1. *Michel*. A complete absence of the inner ear and auditory nerve. This dysplasia is relatively rare. The person with a Michel dysplasia has absolutely *no* residual hearing.
2. *Mondini*. Incomplete development or malformation of the inner ear, including the osseous cochlea. A child with a Mondini dysplasia might be more susceptible to a perilymphatic fistula or to endolymphatic hydrops.
3. *Scheibe*. Incomplete development, malformation, or degeneration of the membranous cochlea. Scheibe probably is the most common dysplasia.

Synergistic Effects

Synergistic means that two or more conditions that occur together may increase or magnify the effect. For example, a low-birth-weight baby may have some but not considerable difficulty breathing. The neonate may be placed in an incubator that has safe noise levels but has some associated noise and impulse sounds. In addition, he or she might be given medication, perhaps a mycin drug for suspected infection, but in doses known to be safe and not associated with ototoxicity. Each condition by itself holds no or minimal risk for hearing impairment, but together, the synergistic effect of multiple conditions can cause a hearing impairment.

Synergistic effects are unpredictable and difficult to prove in a given child. Nevertheless, when taking a case history, it is important to recognize that risk factors can act together to produce a result that each alone is unlikely to cause.

Auditory Neuropathy

Neuropathy is defined as a disease of the nervous system. Auditory neuropathy, therefore, is a disease or disorder of the auditory neural system, including the VIIIth cranial nerve (auditory nerve), brainstem, and cortical pathways. This term typically does not refer to tumors; some auditory neuropathies may be caused by a genetic disorder but many others are idiopathic, which means that their cause is unknown. Some patients also have sensory (cochlear) hearing losses, making neuropathy difficult to diagnose. Most patients with auditory neuropathy have a hearing loss that shows up on the audiogram, and the audiometric configuration could be flat or rising with absent acoustic reflexes. The hearing loss may progress, improve, or fluctuate. The ability to recognize words generally is poorer than would be expected based on patients' pure-tone thresholds. The patient typically has normal otoacoustic emissions (OAEs) but auditory brainstem responses (ABRs) are absent (Berlin, 1998; Hood, 1998).

The definition, description, and management of auditory neuropathies are controversial. Some professionals suggest that the patient NOT be amplified in order to protect the hair cells in the cochlea, while others recommend trying FM systems or compression hearing aids. Sometimes, cochlear implants or vibrotactile devices are considered. Overall, these children many not do well with amplification because, to return to the computer analogy, their hearing problem is in the "hard drive" and not in the "keyboard." Nevertheless, because the auditory centers of the brain are so critical, every effort should be made to provide auditory input.

Mixed Hearing Impairments

A mixed hearing impairment means that an infant or toddler has two or more ear pathologies that exist at the same time, causing both conductive and sensorineural hearing impairments. For example, a child could have a congenital sensorineural hearing impairment, which is genetic in nature, and also have ear infections. The child's hearing impairment would be the sum of the individual conductive and sensorineural components, and both would need to be identified and managed. Another child might have stenotic ear canals that are blocked by wax, a cholesteatoma (tumor in the middle ear), and a sensorineural hearing impairment caused by anoxia (lack of oxygen at birth). Because a child has one pathology, or one type of hearing impairment, does not imply that he or she cannot have another.

An unfortunate problem is that conductive hearing impairments often obscure coexisting sensorineural hearing impairments (Ruben & Math, 1978). For example, once a child is diagnosed with otitis media, the ear infection often is thought to cause the entire hearing problem. A careful hearing test should identify all locations in the auditory system where a pathology occurs (Hayes & Northern, 1996).

Once an audiologist identifies the type(s) of hearing impairments, a physician diagnoses the specific causes. The physician can then provide appropriate medical management for conductive hearing impairments through medication and/or surgery. The audiologist provides audiologic/educational management including appropriate fitting and use of hearing aids and other hearing technology and habilitative treatment in the form of auditory (listening) training and parent/professional counseling about hearing impairment (Berg, Blair, Viehweg, & Wilson-Vlotman, 1986; Johnson, Benson, & Seaton, 1997).

Progressive Hearing Impairments

Some hearing impairments remain relatively stable; others get worse over time. A hearing impairment that gets worse is said to be progressive.

Causes of progressive hearing losses include large vestibular aquedect, perilymphatic fistula, cytomegalovirus, meningitis, congenital syphilis, ototoxicity, endolymphatic hydrops, autoimmune disorders, delayed hereditary hearing losses, and unknown causes (Pappas, 1998). Any time a hearing impairment is suspected to be progressing, an immediate medical referral to an ear specialist is needed. A CT scan can assist a medical diagnosis. If the cause of the progression can be identified, medical treatment may halt or slow the progressive hearing impairment.

Central and Functional Hearing Impairments

There are two additional categories of auditory disorders: central auditory processing and functional.

A *functional auditory disorder* is not really a hearing impairment. Rather, a child may report a nonexistent hearing impairment or exaggerate an existing hearing impairment. Children sometimes do this as a call for help or a bid for attention. The child might think, "How can they expect me to do well in school if I cannot hear the teacher?" A professional misdiagnosis might identify a child's behaviors as resulting from hearing impairment when no hearing impairment exists.

A *central auditory processing disorder* (CAPD) also is not really a hearing impairment relative to impairment of reception and reduced hearing sensitivity. Instead, a central auditory problem causes difficulty understanding the meaning of incoming sounds. As early as 1954, Myklebust described a child who experienced a central auditory problem as one who could "hear," but who could not structure his or her auditory world and select sounds that are immediately relevant.

Congenital brain damage, head trauma, and stroke are examples of pathologies that can cause problems understanding what is being said, even though sensorineural and conductive hearing is normal.

When a child does not react to sounds, an audiologist needs to determine whether the lack of response is (a) a function of not detecting the sound (peripheral hearing impairment); (b) not being able to interpret the meaning of the sound that is "heard" normally (central auditory processing problem), or (c) a combination of these problems.

Some alerting signs and symptoms for possible central auditory problems include (Chermak & Musiek, 1997; Jerger, 1984):

1. Normal audiogram but difficulty on tests of speech perception;
2. Parent, clinician, or teacher report that the child does not seem to hear consistently;
3. The baby or child makes mistakes in sound localization;
4. The baby or child appears to become confused when several people are talking or when noise is present;
5. The child appears to have more problems understanding speech directed to one ear than the other.

■ INDICATORS THAT PLACE AN INFANT OR CHILD AT RISK FOR HEARING PROBLEMS

In 1994 the Joint Committee on Infant Hearing endorsed the goal of **universal** infant screening and **universal** detection of infants with hearing loss as soon as possible. All infants should be identified before 3 months of age and receive intervention by 6 months of age. If risk factor screening is used rather than universal screening, only 50% of infants with hearing loss will be identified (Parving, 1993). Missing the remaining 50% results in unacceptably late diagnosis and intervention. See Tables 3–1 and 3–2 for a list of indicators from the 1994 position statement.

Additional indications that an infant or child might be experiencing hearing difficulty, or more difficulty than usual, include—

☐ Noncompliant behavior;
☐ Responding inconsistently or inappropriately to environmental sounds or spoken communication;

TABLE 3–1. Risk Criteria for Neonates (Birth–28 Days) When Universal Screening Is Not Available

1. Family history of hereditary childhood sensorineural hearing loss.

2. In utero infection, such as cytomegalovirus, rubella, syphilis, herpes, and toxoplasmosis.

3. Craniofacial anomalies, including those with morphologic abnormalities of the pinna and ear canal.

4. Birth weight less than 1500 grams (3.3 lb).

5. Hyperbilirubinemia at a serum level requiring exchange transfusion.

6. Ototoxic medications, including but not limited to the aminoglycosides, used in multiple courses or in combination with loop diuretics.

7. Bacterial meningitis.

8. Apgar scores of 0–4 at 1 minute or 0–6 at 5 minutes.

9. Mechanical ventilation lasting 5 days or longer.

10. Stigmata or other findings associated with syndrome known to include a sensorineural and/or conductive hearing loss.

Source: From "Joint Committee on Infant Hearing 1994 Position Statement," by Joint Committee on Infant Hearing, 1994. *Auditory Today, 6*(6), 6–9.

□ Preferring loud volume on audio equipment or placing ear on a loudspeaker or on the mouth of a person who is speaking;

□ Turning head to one side to hear better;

□ Withdrawal from activities—appearing "disconnected" from surrounding events;

□ Appearing to be in discomfort in or confused by noisy situations.

Following are some symptoms that a child who is experiencing ear infections might display:

□ Irritability—the most common symptom;

□ Any of the previously listed six factors;

□ Pulling at the ear;

□ Head shaking or banging;

□ Discharge from the outer ear;

□ General symptoms of illness such as fever, vomiting, disturbed sleep, or lack of appetite.

TABLE 3–2. Indicators for Infants (29 Days–2 Years).

Infants With Certain Health Conditions That Require Screening

1. Parent/caregiver concern regarding hearing, speech, language and/or developmental delay.
2. Bacterial meningitis and other infections associated with sensorineural hearing loss.
3. Head trauma associated with loss of consciousness or skull fracture.
4. Stigmata or other findings associated with a syndrome known to include a sensorineural and/or conductive hearing loss.
5. Ototoxic medications, including but not limited to chemotherapeutic agents or aminoglycosides, used in multiple courses or in combination with loop diuretics.
6. Recurrent or persistent otitis media with effusion for at least 3 months.

Infants Who Require Periodic Monitoring of Hearing

Some newborns and infants may pass initial hearing screening but require periodic monitoring of hearing to detect delayed-onset sensorineural and/or conductive hearing loss. Infants with these indicators require hearing evaluation at least every 6 months until age 3 years and at appropriate intervals thereafter. Indicators associated with delayed onset sensorineural hearing loss include:

1. Family history of hereditary childhood hearing loss.
2. In utero infection, such as cytomegalovirus, rubella, syphilis, herpes, or toxoplasmosis.
3. Neurofibromatosis Type II and neurodegenerative disorders.

Indicators associated with conductive hearing loss include:

1. Recurrent or persistent otitis media with effusion.
2. Anatomic deformities and other disorders that affect eustachian tube function.
3. Neurodegenerative disorders.

Source: From "Joint Committee on Infant Hearing 1994 Position Statement," by Joint Committee on Infant Hearing, 1994. *Auditory Today, 6*(6), 6–9.

Any concern prompted by any item on these lists of factors and indicators warrants a thorough audiological assessment to determine the status of the infant or child's hearing.

■ SUMMARY

Hearing impairment happens for a reason; there is either disease or damage in the auditory system causing the impairment.

One of the main purposes of a pediatric hearing test is to determine the type (conductive, sensorineural, mixed, central, or functional) and degree (minimal, mild, moderate, moderately severe, severe, or profound) of auditory disorder. If there are several types of hearing impairments, all should be identified.

For more detailed discussions of ear pathologies, the reader is referred to Bess (1988), Fritsch and Sommer (1991), Hayes & Northern (1996), Martin and Clark (1996), Northern (1996), and Pappas (1998).

CHAPTER 4

The Assessment of Hearing Loss in Infants and Children

The primary purpose of assessment is to provide information that can serve as the basis for intervention. To that end, there are several points worth remembering relative to testing the hearing of infants and young children:

1. An infant of any age can be evaluated.
2. A pediatric audiologist seeks to determine a child's peripheral hearing sensitivity (how much hearing is impaired) and the age-appropriateness of his or her auditory behaviors.
3. The pediatric audiologist collaborates with other professionals, such as physicians and psychologists, in determining a differential diagnosis, which is the separation of hearing impairment from other problems that have effects similar to hearing impairment.
4. A test battery approach (using several tests) is employed, consisting of both behavioral and objective (also called electrophysiologic) tests appropriately selected on the basis of a child's developmental age.
5. Frequency-specific data must be obtained. It is important to know not only *if* a child responds to sound and *how* he or she responds, but also *to which frequencies* he or she responds.
6. Multiple test sessions may be necessary.
7. Parents should be included in all hearing test sessions

(especially behavioral tests) and participate in the diagnosis (Clark & Martin, 1994; Moses, 1985). Inclusion promotes parents' acceptance of hearing impairment and helps make them partners in aural habilitation from the very beginning.

8. The pediatric audiologist seeks not only to *diagnose* type and degree of hearing impairment, but also to *interpret* (through knowledge of acoustic phonetics) the potential impact of the hearing impairment on spoken language communication, as well as to *provide* auditory intervention recommendations. The pediatric audiologist bridges assessment and intervention.

The purpose of this chapter is to expand on these assessment issues and to discuss specific pediatric assessment procedures.

■ DIFFERENTIAL DIAGNOSIS

Differential diagnosis is the separation of hearing impairment from other problems that have effects similar to those of hearing impairment. Hearing impairment is not always easy to identify. One reason for this difficulty is that other problems may resemble hearing impairment by showing a similar lack of response to sound and/or lack of speech and language development. Distinguishing hearing impairment from other problems a child might have is not an easy task. Careful case histories, observations, and multiple hearing tests are needed. As discussed by several authors (e.g., Hayes and Northern, 1996; Myklebust, 1954; Ross, Brackett, and Maxon, 1991), an infant or child might not respond to sound as expected, or at all, due to:

1. *A peripheral hearing impairment.* Sounds are not getting into the brain because the child has a conductive, sensorineural, or mixed type hearing impairment. *A peripheral hearing impairment should always be ruled out first, as a primary or contributing cause of a child's lack of (or inconsistent) auditory responses and/or difficulty developing spoken communication skills.*

2. *A central auditory processing problem.* Sounds get into the auditory system, but the brain is unable to interpret efficiently, or at all, the meaning of the sounds,

due to some degree of brain damage. In an extreme case, meaningful sounds cannot be differentiated from nonmeaningful sounds.

3. *General developmental delay.* A child experiences delay or retardation in many areas including auditory behaviors.

4. *Autism.* A child appears unresponsive to most sensory stimuli and was born that way.

5. *Childhood psychosis.* A child displays deviant reactions to sounds; these reactions did not appear to be present at birth.

6. *Some combination of any of the above.*

A second factor that may complicate the diagnosis of hearing impairment in children is the phenomenon of sensory deprivation. *Sensory deprivation* is a lack of sensory stimulation to the brain due to a hearing impairment which can cause delayed and/or deviant behaviors. As mentioned in Chapter 1, hearing functions on the primitive and signal warning levels as well as on the symbolic level. A peripheral hearing impairment can eliminate the auditory background as well as deny a child access to biological sounds. This lack of sensory input to the auditory centers of the brain can cause a child to demonstrate delayed and/or atypical behaviors that may resemble other developmental problems. For example, a 16-month-old girl was referred for a hearing test. She did not yet walk or make any speech sounds, would not make eye contact, and wanted only to nurse and touch her mother's clothing. She was completely unresponsive to sound and there was a family history of childhood hearing impairment. Multiple behavioral and electrophysiologic tests revealed a severe-to-profound sensorineural hearing impairment. Following fitting of hearing aids and intense auditory stimulation, her unusual behaviors declined. Professionals initially were uncertain as to the co-occurrence of other developmental problems. However, 2 months after her sensory deprivation was alleviated by powerful hearing aids and auditory enhancement that allowed stimulation of the auditory centers of her brain, the child was walking, listening, interacting, and beginning to vocalize. This is just one example of how hearing impairment does not necessarily manifest itself in a straightforward manner.

A third factor complicating diagnosis is the very *ambiguity of hearing impairment.* Hearing impairment is not "all or none." A child may hear some sounds but not others. Distance from a speaker, background noise, room reverberation, and attention all influence how audible and intelligible speech is for someone with a hearing loss. This ambiguous nature of hearing impairment was confusing to one uninformed therapist who removed a toddler's hearing aids, stating that he turned when his name was called when he was not wearing his hearing aids. The therapist believed that if the toddler could hear his name, he must be able to hear everything, so the hearing aids probably were a mistake. The therapist further believed that the toddler's speech and language delay must be due to causes other than hearing impairment. Although this particular child might indeed have multiple difficulties, his moderate hearing impairment was a significant factor in his delayed speech and language development. His moderate hearing impairment allowed audibility, even without amplification, but not intelligibility of speech sounds. He certainly was not "deaf" without hearing aids, but he could not hear well enough to identify the fine word-sound distinctions necessary for the establishment of competence in spoken communication; he could not hear details.

Making an accurate differential diagnosis of hearing loss in children, therefore, is not a simple matter. Other problems can present with symptoms similar to hearing impairment as well as coexist with hearing impairment. In addition, sensory deprivation can cause the hearing impairment to appear to be more than a simple lack of response to sound. Finally, the ambiguity of hearing impairment relative to type and degree, stability, noise, and distance can cause misinterpretation of a child's auditory responsiveness.

■ BASIC AUDIOMETRIC CONSIDERATIONS

There are three main purposes of a pediatric hearing test: (1) to obtain a measure of peripheral hearing sensitivity (rule out or confirm hearing impairment as a cause of the child's problem); (2) to obtain frequency-specific information (test the pure tones that comprise speech sounds); and (3) to observe and interpret auditory behaviors.

To this end, use of a *test battery approach* with children is standard. Several, appropriate, behavioral and electrophysiologic (objective) tests are utilized to determine a child's auditory function. A test battery approach furnishes detailed information, avoids drawing conclusions from a single test, allows for the detection of multiple pathologies, and provides a framework for the observation of a child's auditory behaviors (Jerger, 1984; Stach, 1998).

To ensure accurate results, hearing testing must be performed in an exceptionally quiet place called a *sound-isolated booth*. Testing cannot be conducted in a classroom, therapy room, or physician's office (unless the physician has a sound-isolated booth, such as might be found in an otolaryngologist's office) because any noise can interfere with a child's ability to detect very soft sounds.

An audiometer, a specialized piece of equipment, is used to present controlled and calibrated sound stimuli (see Figure 4–1). If a child will tolerate them, earphones are used to test each ear separately. Supra-aural earphones that fit over the ear have been the standard for many years (see Figure 4–2). Recently, insert earphones have become available and this model has many advantages for testing babies and children (see Figure 4–3). Insert earphones have eliminated the possibility of collapsed ear canals caused by the weight and placement of supra-aural earphones. In addition, insert earphones have reduced the need for masking, and they have enhanced the stability of sound delivered to the ear. Con-

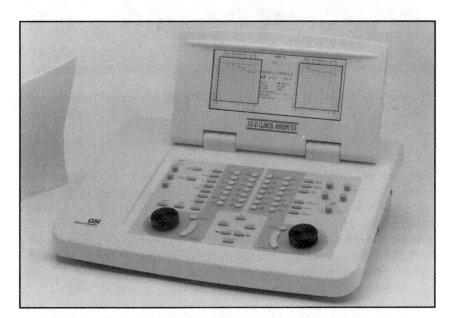

Figure 4–1. An audiometer is used to present controlled and calibrated sound stimuli for hearing testing. (Courtesy of Grason-Stadler, Inc.; from *Clinical Audiology: An Introduction* [p. 196], by B.A. Stach, 1998, San Diego, CA: Singular Publishing Group.)

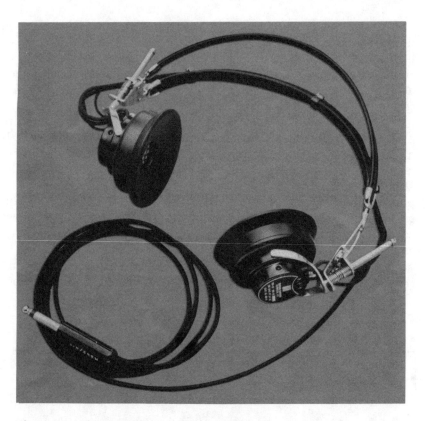

Figure 4–2. Photograph of supra-aural earphones. (Courtesy of Telephonics; from *Clinical Audiology: An Introduction* [p. 199], by B. A. Stach, 1998, San Diego, CA: Singular Publishing Group.)

ditions that would preclude the use of insert earphones include atresia (absent or closed ear canal), stenosis (an abnormally small ear canal), or a badly draining ear due to infections of the outer or middle ear. Although a child may require some behavioral conditioning before he or she will keep the earphones on, most babies and children accept the insert earphones more readily than the heavier, more obvious supra-aural ones.

If earphones cannot be used during a given session, sound-field results are obtained with stimuli presented through the loudspeakers located in the sound room (see Figure 4–4). Testing in a sound-field measures only the response of the better ear; a difference in sensitivity between the ears will not be measurable.

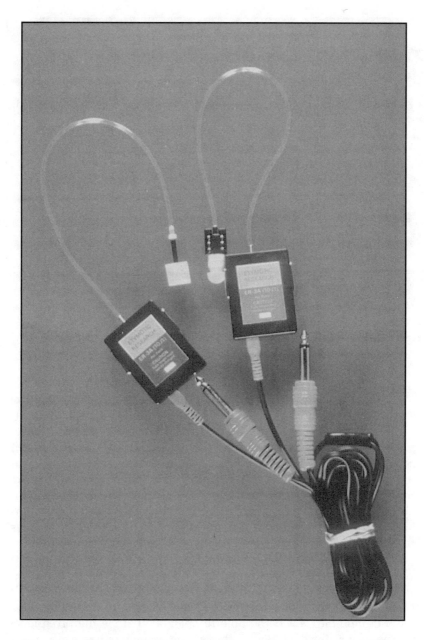

Figure 4–3. Photograph of insert earphones. (From: *Clinical Audiology: An Introduction,* by B. A. Stach, 1998, p. 199. San Diego, CA: Singular Publishing Group.)

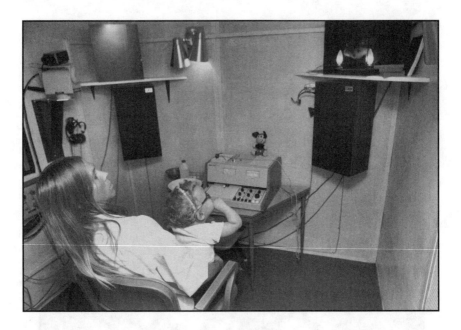

Figure 4–4. For visual reinforcement tasks (VRA), auditory behaviors (usually localization) are rewarded with a visual display.

Measuring a child's responses to different frequencies allows us to study the relationship between speech sounds and test frequencies. The typical tones that are presented in hearing tests are spaced in octave intervals from 250 Hz (about middle "C" on the piano) through 8000 Hz. These particular frequencies are used because, collectively, they comprise speech sounds, rather like individual threads form a cloth (Ling, 1976, 1989, 1997). One is not consciously aware of the individual pure tones contained in someone's speech, any more than one is aware of each individual thread contained in a dress. However, each tone makes a precise and important contribution to speech detection and understanding. If one can detect the low-frequency pure tones (250 and 500 Hz), then one can hear oral-nasal differences, many vowel sounds, and the prosody or melody of speech. If one can detect 2000 Hz, then all consonants, except /s/ and /z/, would be audible. Not being able to hear 4000 Hz, a high-frequency tone necessary for detection of the /s/ phoneme, has important negative implications for language acquisition. For an infant or toddler who is just learning language, missing the /s/ sound means not hearing the concepts of plurality, possessives, first person, and so on.

Clearly, frequency-specific information is vital for interpreting which speech sounds, and therefore which linguistic elements, are audible to an infant or toddler. Use of the Ling Six Sound Test as test stimuli can also assist in this regard, because the six sounds, /a, u, i, sh, s, and m/, are representative of the speech energy contained in all English speech sounds (Ling, 1976, 1989, 1997). Whether a child can detect sound is vital information. Determining the specific frequencies that are detected by a child provides even more important information.

■ BEHAVIORAL AND OBJECTIVE AUDIOLOGIC TESTS

Behavioral audiometric tests are procedures in which a response to sound is elicited and measured, and the function of the auditory system is subsequently inferred. The auditory system is not measured directly. For example, a sound might be presented and the child's localization behavior to the sound source might be observed, with the subsequent inference that the child "heard" the sound. Head turning behavior was measured, not the actual function of the organ of Corti or the auditory cortex; their function was implied.

In contrast, objective or electrophysiologic tests provide some direct measurement of the auditory system—eardrum and middle ear mobility, middle ear muscle reflexes, and neural responses in the lower brainstem. Although objective tests provide some direct indication of auditory function, their results may be open to differing interpretations. Objective tests are *not* tests of hearing.

There is no simple, easy, one-shot method to pediatric hearing evaluation (Matkin, 1990). Multiple tests are used to provide the most complete picture of a child's auditory function.

The next section contains a brief summary of pediatric test procedures, both behavioral and objective. For detailed discussions of methodology and interpretation, the reader is referred to Bess (1988), Hayes and Northern (1996), Jerger (1984), Martin and Clark (1996), Ross, Brackett and Maxon (1991), and Stach (1998).

Behavioral Tests

Behavioral tests are selected based on the ability of an infant or toddler to perform the tasks required. The ultimate and necessary test of hearing is the acquisition and display of behavioral responses to sound. Listed in order of task complexity, from least to most complicated, the tests include: Behavioral Observation Audiometry (BOA), Visual Reinforcement Audiometry (VRA), and Play Audiometry. There are other behavioral tests, such as Tangible Reinforcement Operant Conditioning Audiometry (TROCA) and Puppet in Window Illuminating (PIWI), but they are not in common use (Fulton & Lloyd, 1975).

It is advisable to use the highest developmental procedure a child is capable of performing, due to the potential for obtaining more precise results through strong stimulus-response conditioning bonds. The tester also must be mindful of appropriate positioning of the baby or child during the test session to allow the child to display a variety of response behaviors. Appropriate positioning is especially important for a child who experiences motoric disabilities. Finally, parents should be included in test sessions to be present while hearing is assessed (Clark & Martin, 1994; Moses, 1985).

Behavioral Observation Audiometry (BOA)

BOA is the simplest procedure in terms of the child's task requirements. A selected test stimulus is presented through loud speakers in a sound-isolated room and a child's unconditioned response behaviors are observed. BOA is used until a child can be conditioned to a lighted toy reinforcer (VRA), usually about 6 months of age and certainly by 1 year of age.

Child responses to BOA are not obtained at threshold (threshold is the point where the individual can just barely hear a sound 50% of the time) but rather at what is called *Minimum Response Level* (MRL). MRL is the minimal or softest level to which a child displays identifiable behavioral changes, usually considerably above or louder than his or her actual threshold.

There are several concerns, discussed below, in interpreting BOA results: the infant's state, methodology of stimulus presentation, stimulus parameters, specific responses displayed by the baby, and control of observer bias. Each of these areas should be addressed in an audiometric report when BOA is used as the test procedure.

Behavioral state influences responses that an infant or toddler can or will make (Bench, Hoffman, & Wilson, 1974). Behavioral state is the physical level of awareness of the child. Examples of varying states include deeply sleeping, lightly sleeping, quiet awake and awake active, fussy, crying, and so forth. If a baby is deeply asleep, he or she can respond only to very loud sounds and then with reflexive behaviors such as a startle or limb movement (Flexer & Gans, 1985, 1986). This does not mean that he or she cannot respond to softer signals. If a baby is quietly awake and alert, then there is a likelihood of obtaining meaningful, attentive-type behavioral responses to softer sounds. Thus, BOA responses are a function of an infant or child's state, which should be described in the audiologic report.

The *test methodology* used for BOA should be specified in advance to allow for control of stimulus parameters, response behaviors, and observer bias (Flexer & Gans, 1982, 1983, 1985; Gans, 1987; Gans & Flexer, 1982). Prearranged forms can be developed to record the degree of observer certainty as well as to list all observed behavioral changes. It should be noted that clinician (observer) knowledge of stimulus type and intensity biases recording of responses. Observers tend to "see" responses to very loud sounds and "not see" responses to very soft sounds (Gans & Flexer, 1982).

Infants and toddlers with developmental disabilities may have limited repertoires of response behaviors (Flexer & Gans, 1983, 1986; Katoff, Reuter, & Dunn, 1978). Nevertheless, those behaviors can be divided, generally, into reflexive and attentive types (Eisenberg, 1976). *Attentive behaviors*, such as eye widening, quieting, eye or head searching, and localization indicate higher levels of auditory processing. *Reflexive behaviors* such as startle, eye blink, limb movement, sucking behaviors, breathing changes, and facial twitches denote lower brainstem processing.

Response behaviors, however, are not independent of state and stimulus parameters (Flexer & Gans, 1986). For example, when an infant responds to intense sounds, he or she is more likely to respond with reflexive behaviors. If the child responds to softer sounds, attentive behaviors are more likely to be observed.

The statement often is made that neonates are reflexive responders. If one reads carefully, reports typically note that very intense stimuli were used and the infant was fast asleep. If the same neonate had been awake and alert and had essentially normal hearing, it is likely that some attentive type behaviors to softer sounds would be observed.

The Law of Initial Value (LIV) can be used to interpret an infant's behavioral changes to sound as signifying that a response has occurred (Bench, Hoffman, & Wilson, 1974). Such an interpretation means that the auditory behaviors displayed in response to a sound are in the opposite direction of the infant's prestimulus behavior. For example, if the child was moving before stimulus presentation, her or his poststimulus behavior would be in the opposite direction—the child would quiet if she or he heard the sound. If the child was very quiet before the sound then her or his activity would increase after the sound, if she or he heard it.

Stimulus parameters including meaningfulness (speech and non-speech stimuli), bandwidth (pure tones, narrow-band noise, broad-band noise), intensity (soft and loud), duration (how long the sound is presented, usually about 2 seconds), and between-stimulus interval encompass other important BOA variables (Flexer & Gans, 1985). The stimulus parameters should be specified in the audiologist's report along with the specific responses observed (see Figure 4–10).

BOA can provide a great deal of information about a baby's auditory ability, information that can be used in planning effective habilitative strategies. MRLs can be obtained to different types of stimuli, including the Ling Six Sound Test (Ling, 1976, 1997) and narrow band signals, to provide some frequency-specific information. Responses can be used to estimate auditory function. Although conditioned audiometric procedures are preferred, conditioning is not always possible. BOA is sometimes the only behavioral test that can be used.

Visual Reinforcement Audiometry (VRA)

VRA (Liden & Kankkunen, 1969) and Conditioned Orientation Reflex Audiometry (COR) (Suzuki & Ogiba, 1961) are the most commonly used visual reinforcement tasks. A child's head turning response is rewarded with a visual display, usually a lighted, moving mechanical toy like a dancing bear or a running dog (Primus, 1987). A complex visual reinforcer with lights and animation is more reinforcing than a simple one with lights only (McCormick, 1993). A baby typically is conditioned to *localize* to a toy every time a sound is presented (see Figure 4–4). Because the baby is older and more mature as well as being awake and alert, auditory responses are elicited to softer sounds than those obtained with BOA—typically within normal limits for normally hearing babies. VRA procedures are used until about 2½ to 3½ years of age when play audiometry generally can be used.

Conditioned Play Audiometry

Play audiometry (Lowell, Rushford, Hoversten, & Stoner, 1956), the most sophisticated pediatric task, demands the active cooperation of the child in dropping a block in a bucket or putting a ring on a peg (see Figure 4–5). Most children are close to 2 or 2½ years of age before they can perform play audiometry consistently. Conditioning may not be possible for some children with disabilities until an even older age. Threshold information can be obtained because the child is now mature enough to employ active listening strategies and to maintain attention to task.

Specific speech tests also can be performed. Speech tests evaluate varying levels of auditory skills and are described in Chapter 7 of this book.

The most difficult response task is the **hand raising or button pushing response used by adults**. Some 3-year-olds and virtually every child 5 years and older can raise his or her hand. However, in a relatively long test session where each ear is tested twice (by air and bone conduction), operant and social reinforcement can help maintain attention.

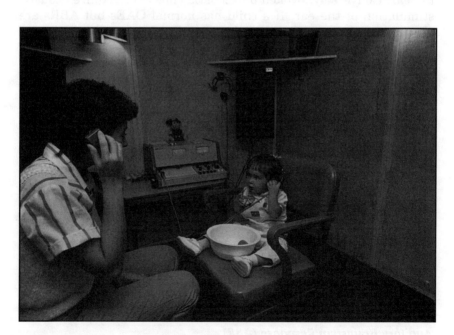

Figure 4–5. Play audiometry, the highest level pediatric task, involves the active cooperation of a child; an auditory stimulus is paired with an operant task, such as dropping a block in a bucket.

Objective or Electrophysiologic Tests

There are three main objective or electrophysiologic tests used with infants and young children, **otoacoustic emissions (OAE)**, **auditory brainstem response (ABR)**, and **impedance audiometry** or middle ear assessment.

Otoacoustic Emissions (OAE)

Recent research has found that the cochlea (inner ear) actively produces energy during the hearing process (Brownell, 1990). These emissions are a normal by-product of the micromechanical actions of the cochlear amplifier that is thought to be situated in the outer hair cells. OAEs evaluate hair cell integrity.

Otoacoustic emissions can be separated into two general categories: Spontaneous and evoked (Berlin, 1998; Lonsbury-Martin, Whitehead, & Martin, 1991). Spontaneous emissions can be detected in about half of the persons with normal hearing sensitivity; they occur in the absence of deliberate acoustic stimulation of the ear. Conversely, evoked otoacoustic emissions require acoustic stimulation of the ear. If a child has normal OAEs but ABRs are absent, auditory neuropathy could exist.

To measure evoked otoacoustic emissions, a small probe is inserted in the ear canal, sounds are presented, and response tracings are recorded. There is no discomfort and the child is not required to cooperate beyond holding still. Evoked emissions are present in the ears of persons with normal hearing sensitivity and are systematically reduced or absent in the ears of persons with sensorineural hearing impairment (Lonsbury-Martin, Whitehead, & Martin, 1991).

Even though the evaluation of evoked otoacoustic emissions holds promise for testing the hearing of infants and children, more studies are needed. The procedure also has limitations. For example, for otoacoustic emissions to be measured, the middle ear must be essentially normal. Because middle ear problems are so common in infants and young children, otoacoustic emissions need to be interpreted with caution. For more information about otoacoustic emissions, the reader is referred to Berlin (1998), Decker (1992), and White and Behrens (1993).

Auditory Brainstem Response (ABR)

ABR is a safe, noninvasive test that does not require a child's voluntary cooperation. Several electrodes, attached to the top of the head and on or near each ear, measure the very tiny electrical signal caused by nerves firing in response to click sound stimuli presented through earphones or a bone oscillator (see Figure 4–6). ABR is not a "hearing test" per se. Rather, the resulting tracing represents the synchronous discharge of first- through sixth-order neurons in the VIIIth cranial nerve (auditory nerve) and brainstem. If the procedure is appropriately performed, information about the sensitivity of each ear can be inferred from the resultant tracing.

Patients undergoing ABR must be very still because movement can invalidate the test. For young children, therefore, sedation (chloral hydrate) is often administered by a physician just prior to the test (Berlin & Hood, 1987).

Tracings must be interpreted carefully because middle ear pathology can complicate interpretation of results. In addition, damage to the brainstem can affect or obscure ABR responses (Kraus, Ozdamar, Heydemann, Stein, & Reed, 1984). If a child has normal ABR tracings bilaterally, one can be reasonably confident that the child has normal peripheral hearing. However, if the ABR

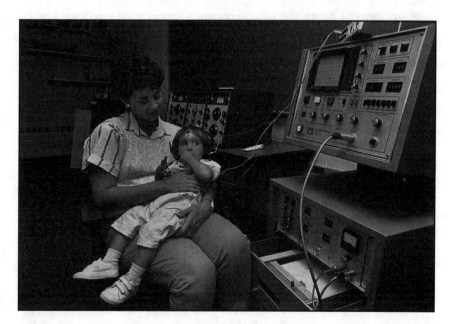

Figure 4–6. Auditory brainstem response (ABR), an objective test, measures the tiny electrical potential produced by the synchronous discharge of first through sixth-order neurons in the auditory nerve and brainstem in response to sound stimuli.

responses are abnormal, interpretation of hearing impairment is more ambiguous (Swigonski, Shallop, Bull, & Lemons, 1987).

When reading an ABR report, the following information should be noted:

1. Were the signals presented by air and bone conduction?
2. Were behavioral tests also performed? ABR cannot investigate auditory behaviors, only behavioral tasks can.
3. Was impedance testing used to look for middle ear problems?
4. Clinical ABR uses tone bursts that correlate most closely with pure-tone thresholds at and around 3000 Hz. Therefore, a child with a sharply sloping high-frequency hearing loss but with normal low-frequency hearing will look the same on an ABR as a child with a flat, severe-to-profound hearing loss. *ABR does not tell audiometric configuration.*

Note that the absence of ABR responses does not mean that there is no residual hearing. Many children who have sensorineural hearing impairments severe enough to show absent ABR responses do have considerable residual hearing that is accessible by amplification technology. The reader is referred to Hood (1998) for more information about ABR.

Impedance (Immittance) Testing

Impedance provides an objective measure of middle ear function. Note that impedance is not a test of hearing. There are three aspects to impedance testing: tympanometry, static admittance, and acoustic reflexes.

In impedance audiometry, a small rubber plug is inserted in the child's ear canal (see Figure 4–7). A continuous tone is presented accompanied by small air pressure changes that cause the eardrum to move. Patterns of eardrum movement and protective muscle reflexes in the ear are measured. Once again, the child does need to hold still because movement affects test results.

Impedance audiometry is a very important part of the auditory test battery because it often provides primary evidence of a middle ear pathology. Tympanometry shows the eardrum's range of mobility from normal, to abnormally stiff, to abnormally compliant (ASHA, 1990b). The ears of infants under 7 months of age may be

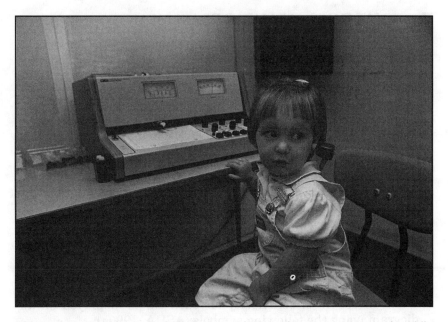

Figure 4–7. Impedance audiometry provides an objective measure of middle ear function, not hearing sensitivity.

too compliant to display accurate tympanometric results (Paradise, Smith, & Bluestone, 1976; Sprague, Wiley, & Goldstein, 1985).

The following points should be considered relative to impedance testing and interpretation:

1. *Impedance audiometry measures middle ear function, not hearing sensitivity.* As such, impedance testing cannot stand alone but must be part of a battery of tests including behavioral evaluations.

2. Middle ear function may not be stable, especially with otitis media. A child may have negative pressure in the middle ear one day and fluid the next. Therefore, interpretation of impedance results really applies only to the *"day of test."*

3. Unfortunately, impedance results are very difficult to interpret on babies under about 7 months of age, unless special equipment is used.

4. Impedance testing, especially for the otitis-prone child, is most meaningful when multiple measures are performed over time, providing a long-range picture of the child's middle ear function.

■ WHAT DOES AN AUDIOGRAM MEAN?

An audiogram is a simple graph that charts what a person can hear. The audiogram is produced by testing a person in a sound-isolated booth using pure tones presented through earphones. This hearing test demonstrates how loud a sound needs to be for a person to just barely hear it.

The audiogram shows the type of hearing loss (conductive, sensorineural, or mixed), the degree of hearing loss (ranging from minimal to profound), and the pattern of the hearing loss (how much hearing loss exists at different frequencies).

Frequencies from 250 Hz through 8000 Hz are shown along the horizontal dimension, and intensity or loudness in dB HL (decibels in Hearing Level) is displayed along the vertical dimension (Figure 4–8). The higher the number of decibels, the louder the sound. Threshold is defined as the softest sound that the person can hear. All sounds greater than threshold (towards the bottom of the graph) are audible. Sounds softer than threshold (towards the top of the graph), are not audible.

The threshold of sensitivity for each ear is displayed on an audiogram using the following symbols (ASHA, 1990a):

1. O = the softest sound that the person can hear with his or her right ear under headphones.
2. X = the softest sound that the person can hear with his or her left ear under headphones.
3. ^ = the softest sound that the person can hear when being tested by bone conduction; the test ear is not specified. See Figure 4–9 for a photograph of a bone conduction transducer.

All of the above audiometric symbols specify that the nontest ear was not masked—removed from the test situation by having a static noise "keep it busy." Different symbols designate when masking has been used. For example, a triangle (△) is used when the right ear is tested by air conduction while the left ear is being masked. An open box (□) is used when the left ear is being tested by air conduction while the right ear is masked. A left bracket ([) means that the right ear was tested by bone conduction while the left ear is masked. And a right bracket (]) means that the left ear was tested by bone conduction while the right ear was masked. Masking is used when there is a possibility that the nontest ear is responding rather than the test ear, thereby contaminating the test results. Masking is then used to ensure that the ear being tested is indeed the ear responding to the test tone.

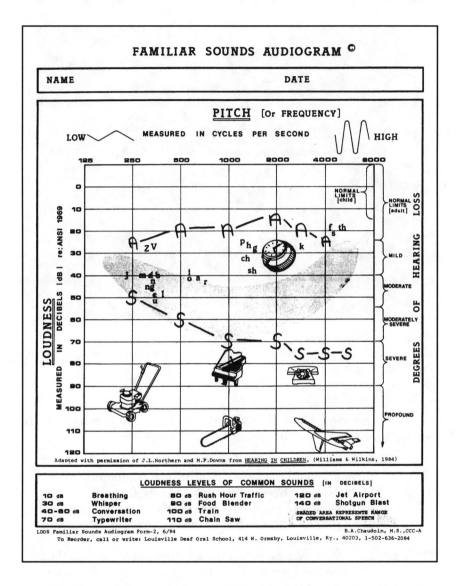

Figure 4–8. This audiogram (graph of an individual's hearing sensitivity) shows not only frequency (pitch) and intensity (loudness), but also the relationship of both to specific speech and environmental sounds. On this audiogram, aided thresholds **(A)** show the softest tones that the child can hear while wearing his or her hearing aids, compared to unaided sound-field thresholds **(S)**, which show the softest sounds the child can hear without amplification. The Familiar Sounds Audiogram is printed with permission of its developer, Barbara A. Chaudoin, MS, CCC/A, audiologist at The Louisville Deaf Oral school.

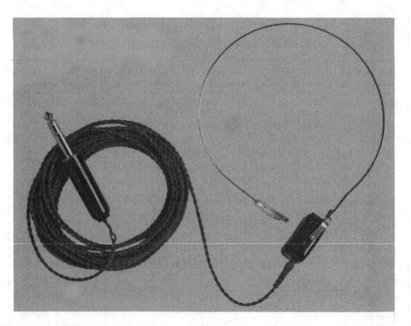

Figure 4–9. Photograph of a bone-conduction transducer. (From *Clinical Audiology: An Introduction* [p. 199], by B. A. Stach, 1998, San Diego, CA: Singular Publishing Group.)

A legend should be included that defines all symbols used on the audiogram. Additional audiometric symbols include:

1. *S = Sound-field thresholds.* The tones are presented through loudspeakers directly into the sound room. Sound-field thresholds often are obtained when a baby or young child will not wear earphones or when a comparison is needed between hearing aided and unaided tones.

2. *A = Aided sound-field thresholds.* The softest sounds that a person can hear while wearing hearing aids. Whenever a child wears hearing aids, sound-field aided measurements must be made to determine how the child is functioning with amplification in the real world. A child's aided sensitivity cannot be known without obtaining data. It is therefore important to include aided as well as unaided thresholds on a child's audiogram to compare, according to acoustic phonetics, speech sounds that are audible with and without amplification.

In the example shown in Figure 4–8, note the relationship between aided and unaided thresholds. The young child depicted on the audiogram has a moderate-to-severe hearing loss as assessed in sound field. Average conversational speech would *not* be audible to this child, but many environmental sounds would be heard without amplification. When wearing her hearing aids, *all* of conversational speech and all speech sounds would be acoustically available—provided that the speaker is close to the child, the environment is relatively quiet, the child is attending, and many meaningful listening opportunities are presented.

This child's amplification (see Figure 4–8) is providing a wonderful "keyboard" through which data can be entered into her brain. What if this child was brought to your early intervention program without the hearing aids? What if the battery "died" during therapy? What if the parents put the hearing aids on her for only a few hours each day? This child has a great deal of very usable residual hearing, *but residual hearing is of no value unless and until it is accessed via appropriate amplification that maximizes the child's ability to hear speech.*

■ OBSERVATION OF AUDITORY BEHAVIORS

Following is a list of behaviors that an infant or child may exhibit in response to speech and/or environmental sounds. It may be helpful to use this form to check off the behaviors that are observed and to note the specific sounds that appear to elicit the responses. It also would be helpful to observe the sounds the child can detect without amplification, as compared to sounds that can be detected *only* when the child is wearing amplification.

Note that background noise, distance from the source, competing sensory stimuli, ability to move, the child's behavioral state, and attention all influence a child's auditory behaviors. Because distance, environment, and infant positioning are controlled during audiologic testing, the audiologist may elicit behaviors that are not apparent in other learning domains.

Attentive Behaviors

These behaviors often suggest learning:

- ☐ If sleeping, the child awakens to sudden noises (arousal).
- ☐ The child is soothed by mother's or caregiver's voice (quieting).

- ☐ Eye widening, a type of "What is it?" response.
- ☐ The infant or child's eyes are observed to search for the sound but the head is held still.
- ☐ Eyes appear to localize directly to the sound.
- ☐ The child exhibits head searching and perhaps a rudimentary head turn toward the sound.
- ☐ The child turns his or her head toward the side where the sound is presented.
- ☐ The child localizes directly when sound is presented to the side, below, and/or above.
- ☐ The infant or child smiles in response to sound.

Reflexive Behaviors

These behaviors typically are elicited at the level of the lower brainstem, thus their presence does not imply learning:

- ☐ The infant or child startles when sound is presented in a quiet room.
- ☐ The child's limbs move when sound is presented.
- ☐ The child's eyes blink when sound is presented in a quiet environment.
- ☐ The child starts or stops sucking when sound is presented.
- ☐ The child's breathing rate changes when sound is presented.
- ☐ Facial twitches, frowns, or grimaces are noted when sound is presented.
- ☐ The child starts or stops crying to loud sounds.

Note that arousal and quieting behaviors may be interpreted as either reflexive or attentive behaviors.

Even if an infant or child initially responds to sound with reflexive behaviors, he or she deserves an opportunity to learn to respond more meaningfully. Current auditory function does not necessarily predict future auditory potential.

■ "UNSCIENTIFIC" OBSERVATIONS BASED ON 25 YEARS OF EXPERIENCE

Following are some summary observations and opinions that the author has formulated during 25 years of experience.

- For infants with multiple disabilities, the assessment and management of hearing and subsequent stimulation of auditory brain centers are a priority that should be accomplished immediately after the baby's life has been stabilized. Do not delay! Early auditory experience is a critical factor in development.
- Observe and ask parents and teachers how the child responds to sounds outside of the audiologic test suite; our audiological results need to be reconciled with the baby's real-world behaviors.

For example, if the child is audiometrically hard of hearing, then some unamplified behaviors to sound ought to have been observed. On the other hand, if the child is audiometrically deaf, then the child would have had no access to unamplified sound, and his or her behaviors should reflect that fact.

- Begin the test session with noisemakers or the Ling 6 Sounds before entering the test suite. Observe the infant or child's auditory behaviors, first unaided and then with hearing aids (if the child wears them).
- If teachers and parents are very unsure about a child's response to sound—the child probably did NOT respond.
- Use insert earphones rather than supra-aural ones; children typically tolerate them best, and more reliable ear-specific thresholds or MRLs can be obtained.
- Begin the audiological diagnostic assessment by using appropriate speech material, rather than pure tones.
- Include a word identification test, or some developmentally appropriate speech test at an average conversational level of loudness (45 dB HL) in both the unaided and aided conditions to evaluate FUNCTIONAL ability.
- Use warble tones instead of pure tones to obtain frequency-specific data; they are easier to hear and more interesting to babies and children. Narrowband noise, the Ling 6 Sounds, or both can be used to get some frequency specificity if the child does not respond well to warble tones.
- When testing with warble tones or narrowband noise, begin testing at 250 Hz (low frequencies) rather than at 1000 Hz, especially if the child has a history of anoxia.

- Include 12,000 Hz to obtain a more complete idea about audiometric configuration; is there a saucer-shaped pattern to the hearing loss?
- When testing a child, closely observe all of the behavioral changes displayed by the child when you are certain that the child responded or was well-conditioned to a task. Note facial expression, body tension, "connectedness," and response latency.
- During the test session, if the child stops responding to stimuli, return to a stimulus type and intensity where you are certain that the child responded. (a) If the child again responds, then we can infer that his or her later lack of response occurred because the child did not hear the stimuli. (b) However, if the child does not respond to a stimulus that he or she previously responded to, then we can infer that the child may have habituated.
- Plot all unaided, aided, FM, and cochlear implant thresholds on a "Familiar Sounds" audiogram to assist in parent and teacher counseling.
- If a child has a hearing loss, always try amplification, no matter how severely disabled a child might appear to be.
- For children with severe disabilities, try an appropriately adjusted FM system, whether or not they have a peripheral hearing loss—the remote microphone of an FM system increases the saliency of spoken language by improving the signal-to-noise ratio.
- Do impedance testing last, unless the child is older or you know that the child will not be frightened or annoyed by the procedure.
- Fit an FM system for home use within 3 months of fitting a hearing aid on an infant or toddler—the parents can use the remote microphone of the FM system to expand the child's distance hearing and incidental learning. We are creating an auditory world for the child; and technology is essential for acoustic accessibility in all of a child's environments.
- If the baby or young child has a profound hearing loss (audiometric thresholds 90 dB HL or worse), or if hearing loss appears to be progressive with poor speech discrimination ability, refer to a cochlear implant center for an evaluation.

- Listen to the child's speech or prespeech utterances—a child typically sounds like what they hear.
- An audiologist ought to be able to plot the child's audiogram based on how the child sounds.
- At the first visit to an audiologist, an infant's or young child's development can look very limited due to sensory deprivation, but that same child could end up functioning at a much higher level than we would initially predict. Therefore, beware of letting the child's initial state limit the future prognosis, especially if he or she has multiple disabilities.
- Never rule out hearing as a viable input channel, and do resist the tendency to bypass hearing in the chain of intervention.
- Because of how human beings are neurologically programmed, hearing (auditory stimulation of critical brain centers) could be a child's most powerful modality for growth of communication skills and for being connected to the world.
- Have high expectations! No one knows what is "inside" of a child! There is always hope!!
- As Mark Ross, a well-respected audiologist, has repeatedly stated, the quality and integrity of the audiologic management that a child receives from the beginning are probably the most important factors in determining whether a child will be functionally hard of hearing or functionally deaf.

■ INFORMATION THAT A TEACHER, CLINICIAN, OR PARENT SHOULD REQUEST FROM AN AUDIOLOGIST

The following two forms (Figures 4–10 and 4–11), adapted from Flexer and Baumgarner (1990), specify the audiologic information that would be most helpful in early intervention programming.

The form presented in Figure 4–10 can be sent prior to the child's audiologic appointment or taken to the audiologist at the time of the child's appointment. The information requested on the form is designed to assist the audiologist in providing meaningful audiometric data to the intervention team.

Dear Audiologist:

Please provide us with the following information that will be used to plan educational programming for the child. Send the form to _____

at_____.

Thank you.

DATE: _____ AUDIOLOGIST: _____

CHILD: _____

1. Which audiologic tests were attempted (A) and completed (C)?

    ___Behavioral Observation Audiometry (BOA)

    ___Visual Reinforcement Audiometry (VRA)

    ___Conditioned Play Audiometry (CPA)

    ___Auditory Brainstem Response (ABR)

    ___Otoacoustic Emissions (OAE)

    ___Tympanometry

    ___Static compliance

    ___Acoustic reflexes

2. If Auditory Brainstem Response (ABR) testing and/or OAE testing were performed, how do these results compare with behavioral observation tests?_____

    _____

3. If Behavioral Observation Audiometry was performed, please answer the following:

(continued)

Figure 4–10. Information to obtain from the audiologist. (Adapted from Flexer, C., & Baumgartner, J. [1990]. Guidelines for determining functional hearing in school-based settings. In M. J. Wilcox [Ed.], *Children with dual sensory impairment series*. Tallmadge, OH: Family Child Learning Center)

a. Stimulus types:

___speech (meaningful signals)

___broad band sound (noise signals)

___narrow band sound (noise signals)

b. To which stimuli was the child most responsive, and at what intensities? _____

_____

c. What was the state of the child during testing? (e.g., awake and quiet, fussy, sleepy)_____

_____

d. Did the child stop responding after a few trials?

____yes   ____no

e. How was observer bias controlled? (e.g., Were "catch trials" used?) _____

_____

f. How many sessions were needed to complete BOA testing?_____

4. Estimate of hearing sensitivity *(air conduction):
   Pure Tone Average (PTA)

   right ear: _____

   left ear: _____

   Does one ear appear to be better than the other?

   ____yes ____no   If yes, which ear?____right ____left

*Peripheral hearing is considered to be normal (on the day of test) if the child responds at *15dB HL* or better at all frequencies in both ears, and if middle ear function is normal as determined by immittance testing.

(continued)

Figure 4–10. *(continued)*

5. Was there an air-bone gap? ____yes ____no

   If so, at what frequencies?_____

   _____

6. How did the child respond to speech? (Please also list/ describe specific words and sounds):_____

   _____

7. What specific auditory behaviors (e.g., startle, localization) were displayed to different types and intensities of stimuli?_____

   _____

   How do these behaviors relate to the child's chronological and functional age?_____

8. How did child respond when the Ling Six Sound Test was presented?

   ah: _____

   ee: _____

   oo: _____

   ss: _____

   sh: _____

   m: _____

9. Which sounds (e.g., vowels, melody of speech, consonants) should the child be able to detect as a function of distance from the child's ears or microphone? _____

   _____

   _____

10. Did immittance testing indicate a possible middle ear pathology?   ____yes ____no

(continued)

11. If the child wears hearing aids, include make, model number, and setting information: _____

_____

_____

Is there an estimate of aided thresholds across frequencies? (Please include aided thresholds on audiogram, if possible) _____

_____

_____

Which speech sounds can the child detect with the hearing aids on?_____

_____

Please compare aided and unaided hearing sensitivity for speech. _____

_____

12. Which of the following assistive listening devices would be appropriate to enhance the speech-to-noise ratio?
___personal FM unit
___classroom (sound-field) FM amplification system
___hard-wired assistive listening device

13. What are your suggestions to assist the child in developing or enhancing auditory/listening skills?

_____

_____

_____

(continued)

Figure 4–10. *(continued)*

_____

_____

_____

_____

_____

_____

14. When do you recommend that the child return to your
     facility?_____

Please attach audiogram and tympanogram to this form.
Thank you.

■ INFORMATION THAT A TEACHER, CLINICIAN, OR PARENT CAN PROVIDE TO FACILITATE THE MEASUREMENT OF HEARING

The information contained in the form presented in Figure 4–11
can provide valuable information to the audiologist about the history and auditory behaviors of the baby or child to be tested.

Parents, teachers, speech-language pathologists, and other
individuals who are familiar with the child can complete this form
and send it to the audiologist prior to the child's appointment for
an audiologic evaluation. Note that the information in Figure 4–11
is presented in addition to typical case history information.

DATE:_____

To Whom it May Concern:

_____has an appointment for an
audiological evaluation at your facility on_____. We
hope that the following information is useful to you. Please
call us if you have any questions.

Parent or guardian: _____

Telephone:_____

Teacher/other: _____

Telephone:_____

Do I think this child can hear? Why? _____

_____

Results of previous behavioral testing: _____

_____

Results of previous Auditory Brainstem Response (ABR) testing:

_____

_____

Results of previous Otoacoustic Emission (OAE) testing:_____

_____

Results of previous immittance or impedance testing: _____

_____

Suspected causes of hearing impairment (e.g., specific diagnosis, history of chronic middle ear infections, excessive ear wax):

_____

(continued)

Figure 4–11. Information *for* the audiologist. (Adapted from Flexer, C., &
Baumgartner, J. [1990]. Guidelines for determining functional hearing in
school-based setting. In M. J. Wilcox [Ed.], *Children with dual sensory impairment series*. Tallmadge, OH: Family Child Learning Center)

Figure 4–11. *(continued)*

COMMUNICATION LEVEL OF CHILD

_____ Does not appear to understand spoken directions, but does follow directions if given gestures.

_____ Expresses needs mostly with gestures and sounds.

_____ Expresses needs with 10 or fewer single symbols (words, signs, symbols on a communication board).

_____ Usually expresses needs with symbols (words, signs, symbols on a communication board).

_____ It is usually not possible to understand child's communication.

Simple one-word commands and object/person names that the child understands (e.g., waves "bye," points to body parts, understands name): _____

_____

Child ____ does/____does not imitate sounds. If yes, what type of sounds? (e.g., car sound, animal sounds, speech sounds, words):_____

_____

MOTOR ABILITIES

The following movements are used voluntarily (e.g., turn head, reach, reach and push, point, eye movement): _____

_____

VISUAL ABILITY

_____ Light/dark perception

_____ Can see only in some visual fields

_____ Sees better when items are very near

_____ Sees better when items are far away

_____ Can see near and far in all visual fields

(continued)

AUDITORY BEHAVIORAL RESPONSES

The following is a checklist of auditory behaviors that have been observed at home or in the classroom:

A. Behaviors observed when loud sound is presented in a quiet room:

_____Startle

_____Involuntary movement of arms and/or legs

_____Blinks

_____Other (please describe): _____

B. Behaviors observed when sound is presented:

_____Change in breathing rate

_____Facial twitches, grimaces, frowns

_____Arouses

_____Quiets

_____Starts or stops crying to loud sounds

_____If sleeping, awakens to sudden noises

_____Is soothed by mother's or caregiver's voice (quieting)

_____Eye widening occurs

_____Searches for sound with eyes

_____Eyes appear to directly localize to sound

_____Head movement as a search for sound

_____Head turn toward the sound

_____Head movement toward sound when presented from different directions

_____Other (please describe): _____

Child is *most* responsive to the following sounds:_____

_____

(continued)

Figure 4–11. *(continued)*

The following are voluntary or involuntary consistent responses to sound:_____

_____

Does child tolerate wearing supra-aural earphones? ____yes ____no

Does child tolerate wearing insert earphones? ____yes ____no

Has the child resisted previous audiological testing? ____yes ____no If yes, how can resistance be avoided? (e.g., audiologist shouldn't wear a white lab coat):_____

Does child respond better to a quiet and subdued or an animated style of interaction? _____

_____

Please list all amplification devices (e.g., hearing aid, auditory trainer) formerly or currently used:_____

_____

How does child respond to the devices? (e.g., resists, is indifferent, cries): _____

_____

Describe how the child hears when wearing amplification devices, as compared to behaviors observed when he or she is not wearing amplification. _____

_____

CHAPTER 5

Technological Management of Hearing and of Hearing Loss

Sound must be detected before auditory comprehension can occur in the brain. Once it has been determined that a child does not have complete and consistent access to the details of the spoken message, what can we do? What are the steps following the identification of auditory disorders, poor listening environments, or both? How can we move *beyond* diagnosis? Remember, ALL auditory disorders negatively affect the developmental process because they interfere with brain access—there is no such thing as an "insignificant" hearing problem.

All hearing impairments in children involve educational issues; some also involve medical issues. Medical treatment, including medications and surgeries, was discussed in Chapter 3. It is important to remember that some children require both medical and audiologic/educational management, and one form of intervention cannot substitute for the other.

This chapter details the components of technological management of hearing and of hearing problems. *The focus of all environmental and technological management strategies is to enhance the reception of clear and intact acoustic signals in order to access and strengthen the auditory centers of the brain.*

Technology is the key to the successful use of auditory input for persons with all types and degrees of hearing loss, including sensorineural. Unfortunately, some parents are told that amplification technology will not help children with sensorineural (cochlear) hearing losses, a statement that is false. Technology enables persons with hearing losses to hear sounds they could not hear at all without amplification. Indeed, without technology accessing the auditory centers of the brain, a child's development and learning opportunities are being limited.

To facilitate the reception of clear and intact acoustic events, the following must occur: control and management of the listening environment; favorable positioning of parent, teacher, and clinician so that talkers are always within earshot of the baby or child; and consistent use of the appropriate forms of amplification—hearing aids or cochlear implants and assistive listening devices.

■ MAXIMIZING THE RECEPTION OF CLEAR AND INTACT (SPEECH) SOUNDS

Sounds must pass to the brain through the auditory system before a child can learn the meaning of sounds. A hearing impairment prevents, in varying degrees, certain sounds from having access to the brain.

Because, as Mark Ross has explained, the main problem with hearing impairment is that one has problems hearing, the first line of audiologic management is the use of technology to access residual hearing (Ross & Giolas, 1978). Hearing is at the core of the acoustic filter; thus if acoustic events are not received, higher levels of auditory processing cannot be accessed (Boothroyd, 1997; Erber, 1982; Ling, 1989; Madell, 1990).

The Listening Environment

In schools and in many other learning domains including the home and clinic, children often are placed in demanding, degraded, and constantly changing listening situations due to noise and distance from the talker (Berg, 1987). The farther an infant or child is from the sound source and the greater the background noise, the poorer the speech-to-noise (S/N) ratio (Berg, Blair & Benson, 1996; Flexer, 1998).

Speech-To-Noise Ratio (also called Signal-to-Noise Ratio)

The *S/N ratio* is the relationship between the primary speech or input signal and background noise. Background noise is anything and everything that interferes with the reception of the desired auditory signal and includes other talkers, heating or cooling systems, home and classroom sounds, traffic noise, computer hums, internal biological noise, televisions, playground, and hallway noise, wind, and so forth. The more favorable the S/N ratio (the louder the desired auditory signal relative to background sounds), the more intelligible the speech or auditory signal will be for the child. An intelligible speech signal provides children with a better opportunity to learn the word-sound differences that underlie the development of spoken communication.

People with normal hearing typically require an S/N ratio of +6 dB for the reception of intelligible speech. Due to the auditory distortion of the hearing loss itself, persons with a hearing problem need an S/N ratio of +20 dB (Finitzo-Hieber & Tillman, 1978; Hawkins, 1984). Due to reverberation, noise, and changes in teacher position, the average classroom S/N ratio is only +4 or +5 dB, and it may be 0 dB, which is less than ideal even for children with normal hearing (Berg, 1986b, 1993).

Rapid Speech Transmission Index (RASTI)

Sound is degraded as it is propagated across a space. However, the amount of degradation has been difficult to determine because of difficulties relating the physical components of high fidelity sound to speech perception. As a result, the negative effects of a typical learning environment on the integrity of speech probably have been underestimated.

The new Brüel and Kjaer Rapid Speech Transmission Index (RASTI) System was used by Leavitt and Flexer (1991) to measure the effect of the listening environment on a speech-like signal. The RASTI signal is an amplitude-modulated broad band of noise centered at 500 Hz and 2000 Hz which is transmitted from the RASTI transmitter to the RASTI receiver (Houtgast & Steeneken, 1985). The RASTI score is a measure of the integrity of the signal as it is propagated across a physical space. A perfect reproduction of the RASTI signal at the receiver is depicted by a score of 1.0. The question investigated by Leavitt and Flexer (1991) was how much speech information is lost as the teacher's speech travels from his or her mouth to the ears of students who are seated at various locations around the classroom?

To measure the loss of critical speech information at various locations in a typical, occupied classroom, Leavitt and Flexer (1991) obtained RASTI scores at 17 different seating locations. Results showed that significant sound degradation occurred as the

RASTI receiver was moved away from the RASTI transmitter. The magnitude of the loss of critical speech information was reflected by a significant decrease in RASTI scores. Even in the front row center seat, which was the most favorable seat in the classroom, the RASTI score dropped to 0.83. In the back row, the RASTI score decreased to 0.55 reflecting a loss of 45% of equivalent speech intelligibility in a quiet, occupied classroom. *A perfect RASTI score of 1.0 could be attained only at the 6-inch reference position.*

These RASTI scores represent only the loss of speech fidelity that might be expected at the student's ear or hearing aid microphone in a quiet classroom. **The negative effects that the student's central auditory processing deficit, hearing impairment (even a minimal hearing impairment), or attention/listening problem will have on speech intelligibility must be considered over and above the degraded speech signal.**

Even in a front-row center seat, the loss of critical speech information is substantial for a young child who is in the process of learning language and acquiring knowledge. Obviously, the most sophisticated of hearing aids cannot re-create those aspects of the speech signal that have been lost during transmission across the physical space.

The importance of being close to the speaker, either physically or through the use of a remote location microphone for the purpose of obtaining a complete speech signal, was demonstrated by the RASTI study. **As soon as any pupil in the classroom or infant or child in a learning situation moves further away than 6 inches from the speaker's mouth, the speech signal begins to degrade.** Data input precedes data processing. *Thus, if a child does not receive a complete speech signal, that child is being denied access to spoken communication.*

Acoustic Guidelines

The American Speech-Language-Hearing Association (ASHA, 1995) recommended the following acoustic guidelines for classrooms: ambient noise level in an unoccupied classroom should not be louder than 30 to 35 dBA; reverberation time (echo) should not exceed 0.4 s; and the signal-to-noise ratio should not be poorer than +15 dB (anywhere in the room). Unfortunately, most classrooms, including early intervention classrooms and therapy rooms where multiple activities are taking place, far exceed these recommended noise levels (Berg, Blair, & Benson, 1996).

Positioning

One strategy for enhancing the S/N ratio is to move closer to the infant or child's ear so that the speaker's voice will take precedence over all background sounds. Yelling from across the room promotes only audibility (hearing the presence of speech), not intelligibility (hearing differences among speech sounds), whereas an average loudness of speech very close to the ear facilitates intelligibility of the speech signal. Sitting across from a child does not produce as favorable an S/N ratio as sitting next to a child.

A noisy room cannot possibly allow an effective S/N ratio. In fact, typical home and building noises (heating and cooling systems, televisions, lawn mowers, hallway noise, Xerox machines, lawn sprinklers) can interfere with the child's ability to hear a clear speech signal.

If speech is being used as the communication vehicle, then educators and family members must be mindful of the potential intelligibility of the speech signal. The environment needs to be as quiet as possible. Turn off televisions, stereos, videos, food processors, popcorn makers, electric mixers and blenders, lawnmowers, and radios. Position yourself close to the child's ear. *The acoustic characteristics of the learning environment, whether the environment is the home, car, school, store, or zoo, is a learning variable that must be managed to provide the child with an opportunity to receive clear "data input."*

Hearing Aids

Hearing aids—miniature public address systems—typically are the initial technology used to enhance the reception of sound for an individual who has a hearing impairment. Hearing aid styles include behind the ear (BTE) or ear level—the most common and advantageous for children; in the ear (ITE), in the canal (ITC), and completely in the canal (CIC)—not usually suitable for children due, in part, to inability of these styles to couple to assistive listening devices and to ear canal growth; and body worn—once the rule for children, but now rarely used due to new powerful BTE hearing aids.

Hearing aids do not correct the hearing impairment; rather, they function to amplify and shape the incoming sounds to make them audible to the child.

Once sounds are detected by a child, he or she must then have rich, meaningful listening experiences to learn to make sense of the new incoming sounds. Sounds must be audible before higher level auditory skills and development can occur. Therefore, amplification is an initial step in the educational management of hearing loss, but it is not the only step, and it certainly is not the last step (Ross, Brackett, & Maxon, 1991).

Although hearing aids can be fitted on infants of any age, a successful hearing aid fitting can be difficult on infants under 6 months of age due to the following practical issues (Pediatric Working Group of the Conference on Amplification for Children with Auditory Deficits, 1996): (a) parental acceptance of their infant's hearing loss, (b) small ear canal and small overall ear size that causes the earmold fit to be difficult, (c) money issues and funding availability, (d) additional child health concerns, (e) conductive component to the hearing loss, and (f) acoustic feedback. Loaner hearing aids, FM systems with a remote microphone, and specialized devices to help with hearing aid retention such as kiddie earhooks, double-sided tape, headbands, and bonnets could address these practical issues. **The earlier that an infant's auditory brain centers are accessed, the better, due to neural plasticity, so every effort should be made to manage barriers to early hearing aid and FM fittings.**

Appropriate fitting is a complex and ongoing process, but it is crucial to maximizing a child's residual hearing. A fitting protocol that was developed specifically for infants and children is the *Desired Sensation Level Method* (DSL; Moodie, Seewald, & Sinclair, 1994; Seewald, 1992). The general goal of this method is to provide infants and children with amplified speech that is audible, comfortable, and undistorted across the broadest relevant frequency range possible.

The reader is referred to the following additional resources for detailed discussions of hearing aids in general and of specific pediatric hearing aid fitting and management issues: Bentler (1996); Bess, Gravel, and Tharpe (1996); Leavitt (1996); Martin and Clark (1996); Moodie, Seewald, and Sinclair (1994); Stach (1998); Tye-Murray (1998); and Appendix 5-F of this book.

Changing Hearing Aid Technology and Other High-Tech Features

Over the years, hearing aids have become smaller and have incorporated sophisticated design features. All hearing aids on the market today are gain based; i.e., they make incoming sounds louder. Most do a good job, *provided* the target gain or amplification for audibility of the speech spectrum is reached for each frequency (Bentler, 1996). No hearing aid can allow speech to be heard nearly as well in noise as in quiet; control of microphone design and microphone directivity seem to be the best way to hear in noise so far, outside of using an FM system with a remote microphone placed close to the sound source (Valente, 1998).

Following are some terms that describe hearing aid features.

- **Microphone Arrangement—omnidirectional versus directional:** An *omnidirectional microphone* is sensitive to sounds from all directions, while a *directional microphone* focuses on sounds in front of a person and reduces the loudness of sounds from behind the person.

  A directional microphone is more helpful than an omnidirectional microphone when listening in noise, provided that the desired sound source is in front of the listener. Note that directional microphones are not helpful in reverberant environments (e.g., classrooms), and directional microphones could limit a child's opportunities to be connected to her or his environment when meaningful sounds occur from the side and back as well as from the front of the child.

- **Linear Amplification:** The *linear nonadjustable circuit* is the oldest type used in electronic hearing aids. This technology is the most basic approach to hearing-aid fitting and provides the same amount of amplification for all types of sounds, whether they are loud or soft, up to the point of the hearing aid's maximum power. This type of hearing aid does not allow adjustment to better fit the needs of the hearing-aid wearer and is NOT appropriate for children. The *linear adjustable circuit* is a step above the previously mentioned nonadjustable circuit because it allows the audiologist to make some amplification adjustments, usually by means of a small screwdriver. This hearing-aid circuit still gives the same amount of amplification for loud and soft sounds. A linear system can provide 8 to 10 dB more gain or amplification than compression circuits, and the distortion products of linear circuits can add valuable speech-spectrum timing cues for children with severe to profound hearing losses.

■ **Nonlinear/Compression Amplification:** *Nonlinear* means that the relationship between the input sound and the output sound is not proportional. For example, soft sounds are amplified to a greater extent than are loud sounds. *Compression* describes how the amplification of a signal is reduced as a function of its intensity. Compression limits the loudness of sounds so that they are not unpleasant to the hearing aid user.

■ **Programmable Hearing Aid:** A programmable hearing aid is one that requires an external programmer (a personal computer or handheld programming device) to set parameters such as gain (amplification), frequency response, and compression. Most programmable hearing aids provide a great deal of flexibility in their adjustments; however, the hearing aids themselves might not function better than their nonprogrammable counterparts (Bentler, 1996).

■ **Multiple Memories:** Multiple memory hearing aids offer different settings or memories for various listening environments. For example, one memory may be used for quiet listening and another for listening in a noisy restaurant. Ideally, each memory is adjusted to provide the hearing-aid wearer with optimum hearing in that particular environment. A *remote control* often is used to access the different memories.

■ **Multiple Channels:** This feature is a fairly new processing technique in hearing aids whereby low frequencies or pitches are separated from high frequencies, with each of the resultant bands of the signal being processed independently.

■ **Analog Versus Digital Signal Processing:** The primary signal processing strategy used in hearing aids has been analog, which means that the signal is processed in a manner that varies continuously over time. Digital processing means that the signal is represented as discrete numeric values at discrete moments in time. The main advantage of digital hearing aids is the flexibility that results from the ability to program and fine-tune them.

Parents often ask if obtaining the latest hearing-aid design features (e.g., digital signal processing) for their infant or young child is worth the substantial increase in cost. There is no doubt that digital signal processing can improve the flexibility of hearing aid fittings; however, research has not demonstrated that digital processing can significantly improve speech recognition in noise in comparison to analog signal processing (Valente, 1998). Furthermore, although digital is good, there is no evidence that digital is better than conventional, *flexible, and appropriately fitted* technology (Bentler, 1996).

The degree of success that a child exhibits from a hearing aid results from several interactive factors such as the child's residual or remaining hearing; how early the hearing loss was identified; the quality and quantity of auditory-based therapy; the ability of family, therapists and teachers to create an "auditory world" for the child; the quality of the hearing aid fitting; and the use of necessary additional technologies such as an FM system with remote microphone for distance learning and improved signal-to-noise ratio.

The following section provides tips about children's hearing aids and highlights issues to be discussed with the audiologist.

Tips to Remember About Children's Hearing Aids and Issues to Discuss With the Audiologist

- If hearing impairment exists in both ears, two hearing aids should be fitted, one for each ear. Binaural fitting is the rule, not the exception.
- Behind-the-ear aids typically are more appropriate than body aids even for infants and toddlers, because they can use special earmolds and can better attach to assistive listening devices such as FM systems (see Figure 5–1).
- Hearing aids should be worn during all waking hours within 1 month of fitting (if not sooner), augmented by the necessary assistive listening devices.
- Hearing aids should have a strong telecoil and Direct-Audio Input (DAI) for attaching to assistive listening devices (Ross & Leavitt, 1998). A telecoil is an internal hearing aid component. It is activated by an external switch, labeled "T," and it picks up magnetic leakage from a telephone or an assistive listening device. *All of a child's listening and learning environments must be considered when fitting amplification to the child; the hearing aid alone will not be sufficient.*

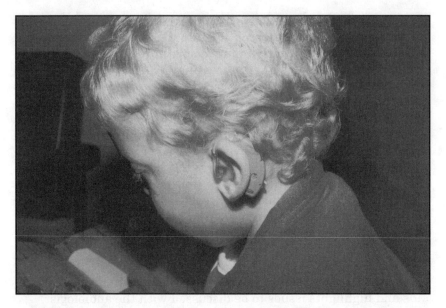

Figure 5–1. Behind-the-ear (BTE) hearing aids, also called ear level hearing aids, are the most common style of hearing aid fitted on infants and children.

- Hearing aids should have internal adjustments for flexibility (tone control to change the amount of low frequency amplification and power adjustments to allow for more or less signal strength). As a hearing impairment becomes more precisely defined following repeated hearing tests, the hearing aid should be able to be adjusted accordingly (see Figure 5–2). In addition, fluctuating hearing impairments need adjustable hearing aids.
- There are waterproof hearing aids that can be useful at the beach and pool. They can be worn during surface swimming, but not for underwater swimming or diving. Some children wear these hearing aids during hot, strenuous activities when they perspire a great deal (see Figure 5-3).
- A listening check must be performed on the hearing aid at least once a day by parents and/or teachers who have normal hearing (Busenbark & Jenison, 1986; Johnson, Benson, & Seaton, 1997). A hearing aid stethoscope should be readily available for this purpose (see Figure 5–4). Hearing aids break, and a malfunc-

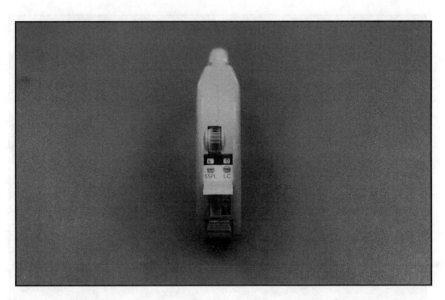

Figure 5–2. This BTE instrument has the internal adjustment capabilities of power output (SPL) and tone control (LC); there is also an external switch to access the telecoil.

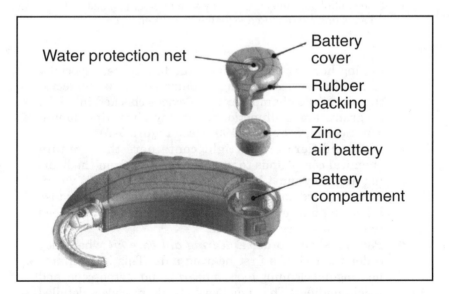

Figure 5–3. A photograph of a waterproof hearing aid. (Photo provided courtesy of Rion)

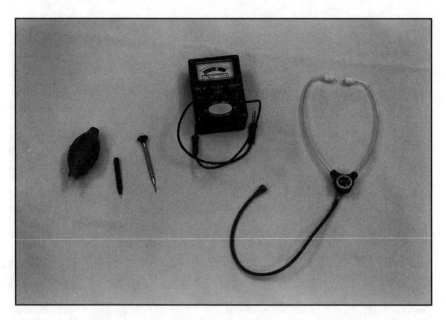

Figure 5–4. Any parent, clinician, or teacher who has an infant or child who wears hearing aids should have the following equipment to check and troubleshoot hearing aids: from left to right, an airblower to clear moisture out of the earmold; a wax remover to clean ear wax out of the earmold; a screwdriver for SPL and tone control adjustments (made by an audiologist); a battery tester (volt meter); and a hearing aid stethoscope for the daily listening check.

tioning hearing aid is of no value to anyone, especially to a child with a hearing impairment. It is no secret that over 50% of amplification devices checked in school programs are malfunctioning at any given time (Johnson, Benson, & Seaton, 1997) (see Figure 5–5).

■ Dehumidifiers are airtight containers that contain chemical compounds to remove moisture from the hearing aid; they must be used to store hearing aids whenever they are not on the child's ear. Moisture can cause a hearing aid to stop functioning, so hearing aids need to be kept as dry as possible.

■ Parents should order a *hearing aid care kit* when they order their child's first hearing aids. This kit contains hearing-aid cleaning tools, a hearing-aid stethoscope, and a dehumidifier. The audiologist should provide a detailed discussion and demonstration of all items in the kit.

HEARING AID CHECKLIST
Visual Inspection
Listening Check

Date:																		
Battery check: (record voltage)																		
Earmold/Tubing Appearance: a. cerumen? b. cracking? c. moisture?																		
Hearing aid appearance: a. crackling? b. volume control c. miscellaneous																		
Ling 6 Sound Test (/u/,/a/,/i/,/s/,$\int$/,/m/)																		
Miscellaneous																		

Key:✔ = adequate; – = inadequate

_____   _____

Figure 5-5. This hearing aid checklist can be used to record hearing aid function over time. (Adapted from J. C. Willis, University of Florida)

- *Hearing-aid brand name* is important. In general, look for the manufacturer that has the longest standard warranty with unlimited repair periods, includes loss-damage insurance as part of the cost for the hearing aid, and provides the most accurate fitting and testing equipment at the best price.

- Battery problems are responsible for the majority of hearing aid malfunctions. Unlike watch batteries, the tiny hearing aid batteries last only a few days to a week in a high power hearing aid. Battery life depends on the power output of the hearing aid and on how often the hearing aid is actually worn.

- Earmolds—custom-made earpieces that direct the sound from the hearing aid into the ear—are crucial to appropriate hearing aid fit (Ingrao, 1997; Leavitt, 1996). Not only must they be comfortable (usually made of soft material for children), but they can be modified to allow better sound transmission (see Figure 5–6). The earmold can shape incoming sound. For example, a horn-shaped earmold will enhance high frequency transmission. An "open" earmold allows some of the low frequencies to filter back out of the ear, as well as letting air into the ear canal, an important consideration if

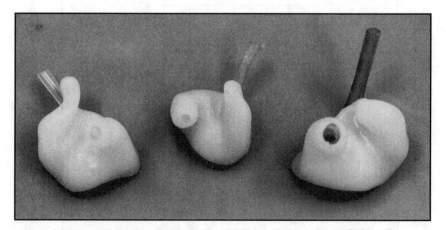

Figure 5–6. These earmolds each have different sizes of tubing and bore openings which shape the sound; the earmold on the far right has "Libby Horn" tubing and a large opening in the bore to enhance high frequency transmission.

the child has ear infections or ventilating tubes in his or her ears. If earmolds do not fit well, feedback can occur. Feedback is that high pitch annoying squeal that comes from hearing aids. Finally, children's earmolds may need to be remade often to accommodate growing ears and to obtain an appropriate fit.

■ Amplification typically should emphasize the high frequencies, if the child has any high frequency residual (or remaining) hearing. The higher frequencies carry the acoustic energy necessary for discrimination of consonant sounds, and consonants are necessary for intelligibility of speech. Low frequencies, however, are also important for suprasegmentals and vowels and should not be deleted. The relationship between low- and high-frequency amplification needs to be carefully evaluated (Ling, 1989, 1997).

■ Visual deviancy and stigma issues should be considered when fitting amplification devices (Flexer & Wood, 1984). Equipment can be fitted in an attractive and interesting manner; harnesses are not necessary. Technology should facilitate, not intimidate, communicative interactions.

■ Aided as well as unaided audiograms must be obtained to provide data about the speech sounds that are audible with and without amplification.

■ In addition to unaided and aided audiograms, real-ear probe microphone measurements should be obtained whenever possible. Computerized probe-microphone hearing aid analysis allows the evaluation of hearing aid fittings through the use of a soft silicone tube that is inserted into the ear canal while the hearing aid and earmold are in place. The resulting analyses enable the audiologist to know the aided response and amplified signal intensity in the child's ear canal (Feigin & Stelmachowicz, 1991; Stach, 1998). The procedure should not cause discomfort, but the infant or child must sit still, and measurement parameters (such as depth of the probe tube in the ear canal) must be controlled. *Note that real-ear measurements should be obtained in addition to, not instead of, aided thresholds plotted on an audiogram.*

■ Repeated aided and unaided hearing tests (including real-ear measurements) and electroacoustic amplification checks should be an integral part of the habilitative program, occurring every 3 months until the age of three (Estabrooks, 1994; Matkin, 1981; Pappas, 1998). Please refer to Appendix 5-F, Suggested Protocol for Audiological and Hearing Aid Evaluation, for more information.

- ■ **If a child refuses to wear his or her hearing aids, check the following** — and then work with the audiologist to fix the problem:

a) *Earmold fit*—the earmold could be too small, too large, or it could rub and irritate specific parts of the ear or ear canal;

b) *Hearing aid fit*—the hearing aid could rub or irritate the child's ear or flop around annoyingly when the child moves;

c) *Hearing sensitivity change*—the child's hearing loss may have progressed so that current hearing aid settings no longer provide sufficient amplification;

d) *Ear-canal or middle-ear infection*—the child may have an infection that hurts when the hearing aid is put on. Medical evaluation and treatment then would be necessary;

e) *Hearing-aid settings*—the hearing aid could be shorting out; it may present sound that is too loud, too soft, or too distorted; or it may provide inappropriate amplification of the speech spectrum. For example, a 3 year old with a mild to moderately-severe hearing loss did not want to wear his newly fitted hearing aids. He cried and ripped them off his ears about 10 min after they were put on. The parents were afraid that the hearing aids were too loud. However, a second opinion revealed that the hearing-aid settings were too soft, so that when inserted, the earmolds and hearing aids functioned like earplugs! The child heard better without the hearing aids than he did with them because he was underamplified. When the hearing aids were adjusted to allow more gain, he not only kept his hearing aids on, he was reluctant to take them off!

Assistive Listening Devices (ALDs)

Hearing aids are not designed to deal with all listening needs. Their biggest limitation is their inability to make the details of spoken communication available when there is competing noise, when the listener cannot be physically close to the speaker, or both. Because a clear and complete speech signal is essential for the development of oral expressive language and reading skills, some means of enhancing the speech-to-noise ratio (S/N ratio) must be provided in all of a child's learning domains (Brackett, 1997; Ross, 1992).

Assistive listening devices (ALDs) encompass a range of products designed to solve the problems of noise, distance from the speaker, and room reverberation or echo that cannot be solved with a hearing aid alone (Berg, Blair, & Benson, 1996; Compton, 1991; Leavitt, 1996; Tye-Murray, 1998). ALDs enhance the S/N ratio to improve the intelligibility of speech and expand distance hearing, thus augmenting a listening function.

There are many categories of ALDs ranging from listening devices (which will be discussed here) to telephone devices and alert/alarm devices (Compton, 1993). The three types of ALDs most relevant to the population addressed in this book include **personal FM systems, sound-field FM (classroom) amplification systems,** and **hard-wired systems**. All ALDs enhance the S/N ratio by improving the audibility and intelligibility of the speaker's voice. Note that an audiologist should be involved in the recommendation and fitting of all hearing aids and assistive listening devices.

FM Unit or FM Auditory Trainer

An FM unit is a personal listening device that includes a *remote* microphone placed near the desired sound source (usually the speaker's mouth, but it could also be a tape recorder or TV) and a receiver for the listener who can be situated anywhere within 50–500 feet. No wires are required to connect the speaker and listener because the unit is really a small FM radio that transmits and receives on a single frequency (see Figure 5–7). Because the talker wears the remote microphone within 6 inches of her or his mouth, the personal FM unit creates a listening situation that is comparable to a teacher being 6 inches from the child's ear **at all times**, thereby allowing a positive and constant S/N ratio.

FM units are the most common assistive listening devices used for infants and young children. For more information, the reader is referred to Compton (1993); Johnson, Benson, and Seaton (1997); Mandell and Sandrock, 1997; and Ross (1992). In addition, see Appendix 5-B at the end of this chapter.

FM units are essential when a child with a hearing impairment, from minimal to profound, is in any classroom or group-learning situation (Berg, 1987; Brackett, 1997; Ross, Brackett, &

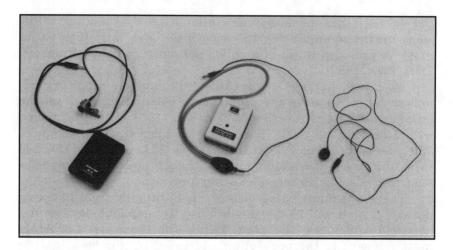

Figure 5–7. A personal FM unit functions like a small FM radio whose wireless transmission of the parent, clinician, or teacher's speech creates a favorable S/N ratio while allowing mobility for both the child and teacher; from left to right, the microphone and transmitter, receiver and neckloop transducer, and external earbud.

Maxon, 1991). Many models of FM equipment are available (Mandell & Sandrock, 1997), ranging in price from about $500 to $2500 per unit.

FM systems can be grouped into two general categories that depend on how the signal is delivered to the listener's ear. A **basic, self-contained FM system (often called an auditory trainer)** typically delivers the signal via a button receiver/earphone; the FM receiver contains an environmental microphone(s) allowing the FM receiver also to function as a hearing aid (usually a body-style hearing aid if the FM receiver is worn on the child's body). A **personal FM system** is similar to a self-contained system except that the child must wear his or her own personal hearing aids to deliver the signal. Please see Figure 5–8 for coupling options for self-contained and personal FM systems.

Recent technological developments have provided the option of a hearing aid and an FM receiver housed together in a behind-the-ear hearing-aid case called a BTE FM (see Figure 5-9). There is no body-worn receiver. Of course, the speaker still needs to wear a microphone transmitter. The child can, by moving a switch, have the unit function as a hearing aid only, an FM receiver only, or as both at the same time (Seaton & Lewis, 1997).

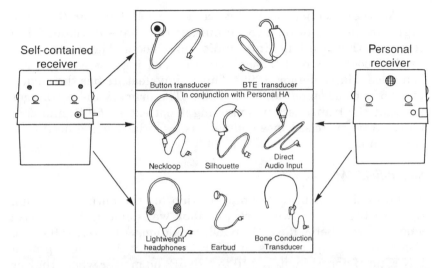

Figure 5–8. Coupling options for self-contained and personal FM systems (Reprinted with permission from "Assistive Devices for Classroom Listening"[p. 62], by D. Lewis, 1994. *American Journal of Audiology.* Copyright 1994 American Speech-Language-Hearing Association).

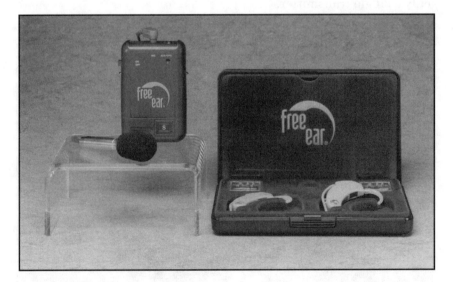

Figure 5–9. Recent developments have provided the option of a hearing aid and an FM receiver both housed together in a behind-the-ear hearing aid case. (Photo provided courtesy of Phonic Ear, Inc.)

Another technological advance is the *FM Receiver Boot* (see Figure 5-10). To date, two manufacturers have developed FM receivers that are built into audio-input boots. These small FM receiver boots can be attached to certain hearing aids when an FM is needed (Hasselberger, 1998). This unique feature has the advantages of a clear signal and small size. The primary disadvantages are that the transmission range might not exceed 50 ft, and care needs to be exercised in avoiding loss, especially when used by a small child.

Sound-field FM Systems

Sound-field units provide amplification for the entire classroom through the use of two, three, or four wall- or ceiling-mounted loudspeakers (Berg, 1987; Crandell, Smaldino, & Flexer, 1995) (see Figure 5–11). All students in the room benefit from an improved S/N ratio of approximately +10 to +20 dB, no matter where they or the teacher are positioned (Flexer, Millin, & Brown, 1990; Palmer, 1997). It should be noted that +10 dB may not be enough for some children with more severe hearing impairments or attention problems; they may need to wear a personal FM unit tuned to the same frequency as the sound-field unit so that the teacher need wear only a single transmitter.

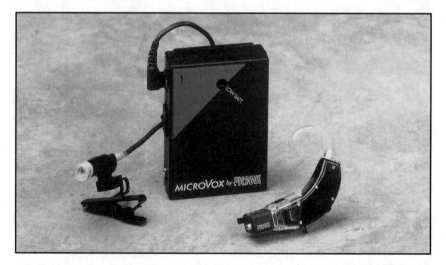

Figure 5–10. Photograph of an FM receiver "boot" for a behind-the-ear hearing aid. (Photo courtesy of Phonak).

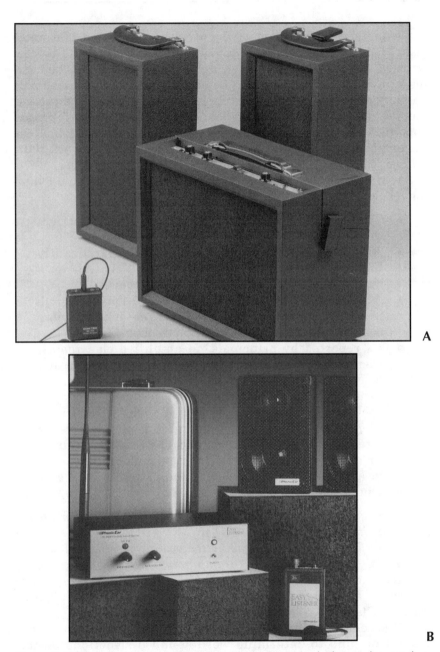

A

B

Figure 5–11. A classroom amplification system is comprised of a wireless teacher-worn microphone/transmitter, an amplifier, and two to four loudspeakers positioned around the room; two different sound-field systems are shown in **A** and **B**. (A is Courtesy of Comtek and Audio Enhancement, and B is Courtesy of Phonic Ear)

RATIONALE. No one disputes the necessity of creating a favorable visual field in a classroom. A school building never would be constructed without lights in every classroom. However, because hearing is invisible and ambiguous, the necessity of creating a favorable auditory field may be questioned by school personnel. Nevertheless, studies continue to show that sound-field FM systems facilitate opportunities for improved academic performance (Crandell, 1996; Flexer, Millin, & Brown, 1990; Neuss, Blair, & Viehweg, 1991; Palmer, 1996; Ray, Sarff, & Glassford, 1984; Zabel & Tabor, 1993). A 3-year study of sound-field FM amplification revealed the following results (Osborn, Graves, & VonderEmbse, 1989):

- The proportion of students requiring special services decreased after 3 years with amplified classrooms;
- Amplified kindergarten classes scored significantly higher on listening, language, and word analysis tests than did children in unamplified classrooms;
- According to formal classroom observations, students in amplified classrooms had better on-task behaviors than students in unamplified classrooms;
- As reported by principals, in amplified classrooms, there were fewer teacher absences due to fatigue and laryngitis;
- Teachers in amplified kindergarten classrooms tended to use less repetition and rephrasing in their instruction;
- The study began with 17 sound-field units; 3 years later, 47 units were in use because teachers wanted them, parents demanded that their children be placed in amplified classrooms, and administrators were convinced that student performance improved.

The logic of sound-field amplification is that, if properly adjusted, it can counteract weak teacher voice levels and ambient noise interference by, (a) increasing the overall speech level of whoever is using the microphone, (b) improving the S/N ratio, and (c) producing a nearly uniform speech level in the classroom that is unaffected by teacher position (Flexer, Millin, & Brown, 1990; Ray, Sarff, & Glassford, 1984; Palmer, 1997) (see Figure 5–12).

If students receive a louder, more intact speech signal, they should be able to determine word-sound distinctions better. Indeed, Flexer, Millin, and Brown (1990) found that nine students who attended a primary-level class for children with developmental disabilities made significantly fewer errors on a word identification task when the teacher presented the words through a

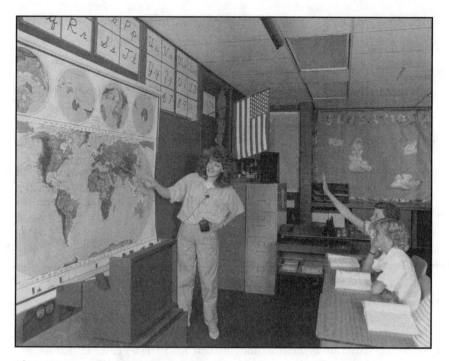

Figure 5–12. The logic of sound-field amplification is that it can provide a favorable and consistent S/N ratio for all students in the classroom. (Photo Courtesy of Audio Enhancement)

classroom PA system than they made when the words were presented without sound-field amplification. Informal observations made during the same study revealed that the students responded more quickly and appeared more relaxed in the amplified condition.

The advantages of sound-field amplification result from the use of a teacher-worn transmitter microphone that is positioned 4 to 6 inches from the speaker's mouth, optimizing critical speech elements. All pupils are consistently closer to the speech source (i.e., the loudspeaker), than they could be to a mobile teacher. The speech signal is not only louder, but each student is closer to the signal (loudspeaker), thereby improving the S/N ratio. However, a pupil cannot be as close to a loudspeaker as he or she can be to a personal FM receiver that directs the sound into the ear. Personal FM receivers can provide a speech signal superior to that provided by a sound-field unit and therefore may be more appropriate for some children.

To summarize, classroom amplification facilitates the reception of consistently more intact signals than signals received in an unamplified classroom, but signals are not as complete as those provided by using a personal FM unit (Leavitt, 1991).

POPULATIONS. There is evidence to suggest that all children benefit from listening to an improved speech signal. However, some children seem to benefit more than others.

The choice of sound enhancement technology depends on the child, the classroom or learning environment, and the needs of other children in the learning environment. Note that a room in a home, a preschool classroom, or a therapy room also can be amplified (see Figure 5–13).

The following populations appear to benefit most from sound-field S/N ratio enhancing technology:

1. Children with ongoing fluctuating conductive hearing losses, primarily caused by ear infections or ear wax, and children with positive histories of otitis media during their *first* year of life. These children required a more advantageous S/N ratio to perform at 50% sentence intelligibility than did their otitis negative peers (Gravel & Wallace, 1992). Because one fourth to one third of typical kindergarten and first-grade children do not hear normally on any given day (Flexer, Richards, Buie, & Brandy, 1994), it seems reasonable to amplify every preschool, kindergarten, and first-grade classroom. The ability to hear word and sound distinctions is a primary basis for the development of academic competencies (Elliott, Hammer, & Scholl, 1989). If young children are at risk for hearing loss and thus learning phonemic distinctions, why not create an acoustic environment that would enable them to consistently and clearly receive intelligible speech?

2. Children with unilateral hearing impairments also will benefit from a sound-field FM system. Some children with unilateral hearing losses may require the more favorable S/N ratio of a personal FM unit, especially if they have major attending problems and language delays.

3. Children with slight permanent hearing impairments (15-20 dB HL) might benefit more from sound-field FM than from a hearing aid in a classroom environment. Once again, depending on the degree of attending, learning, and language problems, a personal FM unit might be more suitable.

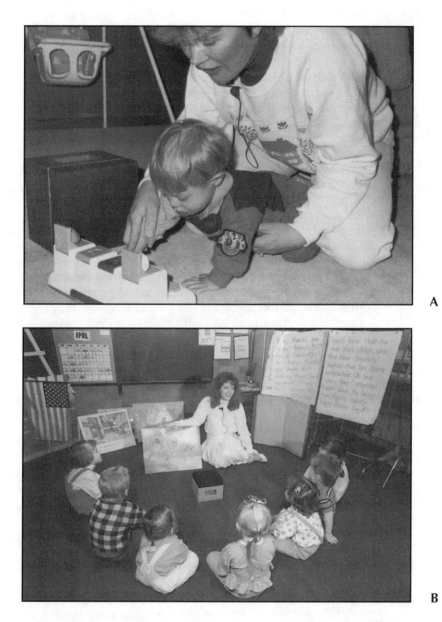

A

B

Figure 5–13. A: A home environment can be amplified using a single loud-speaker; the mother is wearing the FM microphone/transmitter as she provides meaningful spoken communication for her toddler with Down syndrome, who experiences persistent ear infections with accompanying hearing impairment. **B:** A single loudspeaker could be effective for small group instruction (Photo courtesy of Audio Enhancement).

4. Children who have normal peripheral hearing sensitivity but who are in special education classrooms due to language, learning, attending, or behavioral problems would benefit from the increased instructional redundancy provided by a sound-field FM unit. Note that several studies have found that as many as three fourths of the children in primary-level special education classrooms do not have normal hearing sensitivity; furthermore, their hearing problems usually have not been identified nor managed by the school systems (Flexer, Millin, & Brown, 1990).

5. Children with mild to moderate hearing impairments who wear hearing aids might do as well with a sound-field FM unit as they would with a personal FM system (Blair, Myrups, & Viehweg, 1989).

6. Children who have normal peripheral hearing sensitivity but who have difficulty processing, understanding, or attending to classroom instruction could benefit from sound-field FM technology (Chermak & Musiek, 1997). As stated previously, a child with a more severe central auditory processing problem might need the more favorable S/N ratio provided by a personal FM unit.

7. Children for whom English is a second language benefit from the more intelligible signal provided by the enhanced S/N ratio of a sound-field FM system (Crandell, 1996). When one is learning a new language, how much of the acoustic signal needs to be heard in order to differentiate the new words of the language? **All of the signal**...every sound...every word marker; the entire message needs to be intelligible because the child does not have an internal program in the new language that enables her or him to fill in the blanks (Crandell & Smaldino, 1996).

8. Children with cochlear implants also must have the improved S/N ratio provided by a remote microphone (Estabrooks, 1998; Foster, Brackett, & Maxon, 1997).

9. Teachers who use sound-field technology report that they also benefit (Fisher, 1998). Many state that they need to use less energy projecting their voices, they have less vocal abuse, and they are less tired by the end of the school day. Teachers also report that the unit increases their teaching efficiency: fewer repetitions are required, thus allowing for more actual teaching time. One school system noted fewer teacher absences from amplified classrooms (Flexer, 1989).

Three practical advantages of appropriately installed and functioning sound-field FM equipment for target populations are that (a) classroom amplification requires no overt cooperation from the child, (b) the technology is not stigmatizing for any particular child, and (c) equipment function or malfunction is immediately obvious to anyone in the room (Anderson, 1991).

Personal Sound-Field FM Systems

A new type of sound-field FM system is called a personal sound-field unit or Desk Top System (Pillow, 1998; see Figure 5-14). This is a small, lightweight, battery-powered, portable loudspeaker that can be carried from class to class and delivers a clear, close-up sound right to the student's desk. Foster, Brackett, and Maxon (1997) found the personal sound-field FM to be particularly useful for children with cochlear implants.

PRACTICAL ISSUES. There are many issues to evaluate when selecting classroom amplification systems or when recommending a sound field rather than a personal FM system for a particular child, and few data are available to guide these decisions (Crandell, Smaldino, & Flexer, 1997; Flexer 1992). Following is a list of questions that an audiologist should consider in making decisions about classroom amplification:

- What can be done to improve the classroom's acoustics by reducing noise and reverberation?
- Have teachers been given thorough inservice training about the auditory basis of classroom instruction and subsequent rationale for the use of sound-field FM technology?
- What type of microphone should be used: lapel microphone, boom (head-worn) microphone, or collar microphone?
- Who will be the contact person in the district or building to troubleshoot and maintain equipment?
- Will loaner equipment and spare parts be available?
- Is there administrative support for project coordination?
- How many loudspeakers should be installed in a given room?
- Where should the loudspeakers be installed?
- What is the best S/N ratio possible with the equipment?
- What is the durability, quality, and flexibility of the equipment?
- What is the carrier frequency for the radio signal of the unit and the potential for interference (from cellular phones, pagers, etc.)?

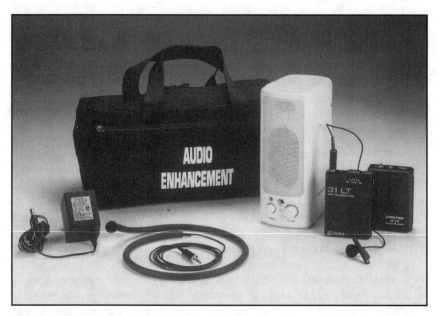

Figure 5–14. A personal sound-field system easily can be carried from classroom to classroom, and the small loudspeaker sits on a student's desk. (Photo courtesy of Audio Enhancement).

- How many discrete channels are available in the frequency band used by the manufacturer? How many units can be installed in the same building while maintaining a good S/N ratio in the equipment itself?
- What is the fidelity of the unit?

SHOULD AN AUDIOLOGIST RECOMMEND A PERSONAL FM SYSTEM OR A SOUND-FIELD FM SYSTEM OR BOTH FOR A GIVEN CHILD? Once we determine that a child has a hearing problem that interferes with acoustic accessibility, the next step involves recommending, fitting, and using some type of S/N ratio enhancing technology. One thing is certain, we cannot manage hearing by not managing hearing. Preferential seating does NOT control the background noise and reverberation in the classroom, stabilize teacher or pupil position, or provide for an even and consistent S/N ratio.

In many instances the best listening and learning environment can be created by using both a sound-field FM and a personal FM system at the same time. The sound-field FM unit, appropriately installed in a mainstreamed classroom, improves acoustic access for all pupils and creates a "listening" in the room. The individual FM system allows the particular child with hearing loss to have the most favorable S/N ratio. The teacher need wear only a single transmitter if the sound-field FM unit and the individual FM are on the same radio frequency.

Whatever type of FM system is selected, the following common-sense tips could facilitate use and function of the technology:

- **Try the equipment.** People must experience FM equipment for themselves; they cannot speculate about function.
- **Be mindful of appropriate microphone placement.** Microphone placement dramatically affects the output speech spectrum. Specifically, high frequencies are weaker in off-axis positions. A head-worn boom microphone probably provides the best, most complete, and most consistent signal. A collar microphone, worn around the teacher's neck, also allows some level of control of microphone distance. If a lapel microphone is worn, it should be placed midline on the chest about 6 in. from the mouth.
- **Check the batteries first if any malfunction occurs.** Weak battery charge can cause interference, static, and intermittent signals.
- **Audiologists should write clear recommendations** for FM equipment, specifying the rationale, type of S/N ratio-enhancing technology needed, equipment characteristics, coupling arrangement chosen, parent and teacher inservice needs, and follow-up visits.

Following recognition and resolution of the equipment-related issues mentioned above comes the realization that, at best, *technology is simply a tool, a means to an end. The purpose of classroom amplification, or any S/N ratio enhancing technology, is to facilitate the reception of the primary speech signal. Once children can detect word-sound differences clearly, they will have an opportunity to develop and improve their language skills and to acquire knowledge of the world*. A 22-minute videotape, "Enhancing Classrooms for Listening, Language, and Literacy," can be useful in conveying these concepts to parents, teachers, and therapists (Flexer, 1998).

The logical next step in the rehabilitative process (see Chapter 7) concerns the child's ability to attend to the now enhanced acoustic signal: listening.

Mild Gain Hard-wired Unit

Several mild gain assistive listening devices are available. "Mild gain" refers to a small amount of amplification. Units with a small amount of amplification are appropriate for children with normal or near-normal hearing. "Hardwired" means that the speaker and listener are connected by wires not by radio or light waves. The lightweight, portable, easily obtained and relatively inexpensive unit discussed in this chapter was assembled from parts purchased at a popular electronics store (see Table 5–1). Specifically, the unit has a small battery-operated miniamplifier/speaker with a 3.5 mm input jack and a 3.5 mm output extension speaker jack with a volume control, a small 360° pickup tie clip microphone, and a Walkman type monophonic (as opposed to stereophonic) headset with a 3.5 mm plug (Sudler & Flexer, 1986; Vaughn, Lightfoot, & Gibbs, 1983; see Figure 5–15). By using a dual mini-phone Jack Adapter, the miniamplifier can accommodate one or two headsets and one or two microphones. Note that some power output is lost with the addition of each headset or microphone; thus the volume setting might have to be increased. Consultation with an audiologist to measure power output is essential before any amplification technology is used. Use of several headsets and/or microphones would be suitable if the clinician had several children in a therapy session, or if the therapist wanted to monitor the sound of the equipment throughout the session. A single microphone also can be moved back and forth from the clinician to the child to enhance both the clinician's and the child's speech clarity.

TABLE 5–1. Materials Needed for One Hard-Wired Assistive Listening Device

Item	Source	Catalogue No.	Approximate Cost
Tie clip microphone, omnidirectional	Radio Shack	33-3013	$24.99
Mini amplifier-speaker	Radio Shack	277-1008	$11.99
9-volt transistor battery for above amplifier	Radio Shack		$ 2.39
Monophonic headset	Radio Shack	20-210	$ 9.99
Dual mini-phone jack adapter (for multiple microphone use if desired)	Radio Shack	274-310	$ 2.49

Note: Based on prices quoted December, 1998.

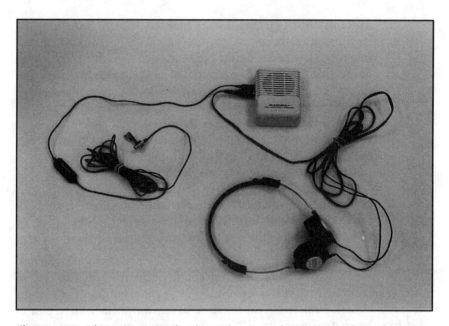

Figure 5–15. This inexpensive hard-wired unit can be used in a therapy situation to facilitate turn-taking skills, to enhance both the teacher's/clinician's and child's vocal clarity (favorable S/N ratio) and to emphasize the auditory modality; from left to right, is the microphone, miniamplifier/speaker, and monophonic earphones.

The most important component of this unit is the external microphone that is attached to the miniamplifier by a wire; the microphone is *not* built into the unit. The value of the external microphone, also called a *remote* microphone, is that it can be moved close to the sound source which improves the S/N ratio.

Leavitt and Flexer (1991) found that the closer the microphone is to the sound source, the more intact the input signal. Said another way, once the listener moves more than 6 inches from the speaker, critical components of the speech signal are lost. Thus, if maximum redundancy is required for an individual to benefit from an acoustic signal, the acoustic signal needs to be as intact and clear as possible.

Several additional issues concerning this simple assistive listening device should be addressed.

1. This hard-wired unit is **not** intended to replace hearing
   aids, personal FM units, or classroom amplification

systems. Rather, this device has the specific function, in limited contexts, of improving the S/N ratio which increases the redundancy of the speech signal.

2. This unit has the limitation of restricting mobility due to the connecting wires between the microphone, the miniamplifier, and the headset; thus it is **not** suitable for classroom instruction.

3. Like all amplification technologies, the unit must be carefully monitored by an audiologist so that power output does not in any way compromise the child's hearing (ASHA, 1991a).

4. Once the appropriate volume setting has been determined by an audiologist, the volume wheel might need to be fixed in position, perhaps with a piece of tape.

Enhancing the input signal (audition) for persons with normal or near-normal peripheral hearing sensitivity through the use of mild-gain amplification devices has been proposed as a treatment strategy (ASHA, 1991a). The logic of using amplification technology has been to improve S/N ratios which subsequently can increase attention span and enhance awareness of acoustic stimuli (Blake, Field, Foster, Platt, & Wertz, 1991; Flexer, Millin, & Brown, 1990). Amplification for the purpose of improving response accuracy by increasing the intensity level of stimulus presentation also has been reported to be effective (Berg, 1987). There are more powerful hard-wired devices too, that are easy to use, such as the Williams Sound PockeTalker (see Figure 5-16).

Following are two examples of children who benefited from the enhancement of S/N ratio by using a mild gain, hard-wired assistive listening device:

EXAMPLE 1: FOUR-YEAR-OLD CHILD WITH MULTIPLE ARTICULATION ERRORS. A four-year-old girl had been enrolled in speech-language therapy for 2 years. Her receptive language abilities were evaluated to be consistent with chronological age development; however, her expressive behavior evidenced multiple articulation errors with severely reduced speech intelligibility. Specific phonological processes noted were deletion of final consonants, stopping, fronting, backing, and cluster reduction. In addition, conversational speech clarity was reduced by a rapid rate of speaking. A lack of progress was noted in therapy and the parents were considering terminating therapy due to problems in motivating the child to attend therapy sessions.

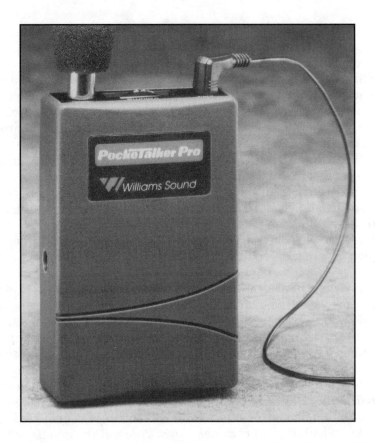

Figure 5–16. Photograph of a personal hardwired amplifier. (Source: *Clinical Audiology: An Introduction,* by B. A. Stach, 1998, p. 508. San Diego, CA: Singular Publishing Group).

A review of audiological data showed hearing within normal limits on the day of test. The parents, however, reported the presence of recurrent otitis media and fluctuating hearing impairment since infancy.

Based on the child's history of early and continuing intermittent hearing impairment, a mild gain, hard-wired assistive listening device was recommended for use during therapy sessions. This device was used to enhance data input through the auditory channel and, consequently, to increase attention to auditory stimuli; the device also served to enhance the child's voice during speech production trials consistent with the goal of improved speech intelligibility.

Comparative data were collected for verbal productions with and without the device. Accuracy of production of specific phonemes was used to document the unit's effect on speech intelligibility. In addition, attending behaviors such as head and neck orientation to stimuli, sitting still, willingness to participate in the activity, and duration of attention to each activity were selected to determine the effect of the amplifier's use on listening and attending behaviors.

When comparing therapy results with and without auditory enhancement, consistently higher levels of accuracy in speech production were obtained with the use of the assistive listening device. In addition, attention to activity increased significantly with fewer clinician cues required to prompt attention. Of critical importance was the parent report of a sharp increase in generalization of target speech sounds to conversational speech.

EXAMPLE 2: INFANTS AND TODDLERS WITH DOWN SYNDROME. Children with Down syndrome often display greater language learning difficulties than can be explained by their cognitive deficits (Miller, 1988). According to recent research, this difficulty in language learning may be attributable to significant ear abnormalities in children with Down syndrome which lead to more than an 80% incidence of continual mild-to-moderate conductive hearing impairment (Dahle & McCollister, 1986). This high incidence of hearing impairment results from (a) stenotic ear canals predisposing this population to cerumen impaction and (b) middle ear and Eustachian tube abnormalities that cause continual episodes of otitis media with effusion.

Clearly, anatomic abnormalities predispose the child with Down syndrome to frequent intermittent hearing impairment that must be managed during early intervention. The child with Down syndrome who may be late in walking also is often visually impaired and depends even more on the auditory system to learn about the environment. Thus, when important data input to the brain from the auditory system is interrupted or distorted due to even a mild hearing loss, the child with Down syndrome is put at an additional disadvantage in language learning.

Continued and aggressive medical management is essential. Equally essential is hearing management provided by the audiologist (Pappas, Flexer, & Shackelford, 1994). Early fitting of hearing aids may be suitable for some infants with Down syndrome who have persistent hearing impairment even with vigilant medical management.

For infants and toddlers with intermittent hearing impairment or difficulty attending to acoustic signals, a mild gain, hard-wired assistive listening device might be recommended for use during infant stimulation sessions (Manning, Flexer, & Shackelford, 1991; Savage & Flexer, 1987). If an infant or child has difficulty tolerating the earphones of the hard-wired unit, a single high fidelity loudspeaker of an FM sound-field amplification unit could be used (see Figure 5–13A).

A center for persons with developmental disabilities used the assistive listening device (in addition to vigorous medical management of conductive pathologies) in an auditory-based program of language enrichment for six infants with Down syndrome. After 18 months of therapy, the six infants had age-appropriate receptive and oral expressive behaviors and were performing at higher levels than six infants/toddlers with Down syndrome who had not experienced acoustic enhancement of verbal input (Pappas, Flexer, & Shackelford, 1994). Note that therapy was not withheld from the six children in the control group. They had not been referred for early intervention, thus they had not been available for services.

Many infants and children across many diagnostic categories potentially could benefit from receiving an improved S/N ratio. Indeed, any infant or child who has difficulty responding to and learning from an acoustic signal of reduced redundancy could profit from access to a mildly amplified speech signal that contains all critical phonetic components.

Audiologists are responsible for recommending, where appropriate, suitable technology and strategies to facilitate auditory function. The mild gain, hard-wired assistive listening device (that uses a remote microphone), discussed in this chapter is one piece of equipment that can improve the S/N ratio, thereby improving attention and performance.

Following trial therapy with the hard-wired unit, client performance data should be obtained to enable the audiologist to justify the additional technological recommendation of a personal FM unit or a classroom amplification system to facilitate a child's education. If a child demonstrates improved attention and superior performance when he or she receives an enhanced S/N ratio in a controlled therapy situation, the audiologist has objective data to support the recommendation of technology designed to improve the S/N ratio in different learning domains (e.g., a mild-gain personal FM unit or a classroom amplification system).

Frequency Transposition Hearing Aid

The TranSonic hearing aid system, developed by AVR (Sonovation) Communications Ltd. in Israel, is designed for persons with a profound hearing loss in the high frequencies and a moderate to severe hearing loss in the lower frequencies. The inaudible high-frequency speech sounds are transposed to a lower frequency region where residual hearing exists, creating audibility of those previously unavailable high-frequency sounds. The TranSonic uses a frequency transposition process that is dynamic and is driven in real-time to respond to spectral changes in the incoming speech signal. The system is very flexible, needs to be programmed by an audiologist, and must be accompanied by an intensive auditory-based treatment program. Some people report very good improvement in sound and speech reception (Johnson, Benson, & Seaton, 1997). This device has been used as an alternative to a cochlear implant for some children.

Tactile Communication Devices

Tactile communication devices analyze sound into frequency bands and convert the frequency bands into signals that are felt on the skin as vibrations from electrical impulses. Tactile aids can be worn on the sternum, abdomen, neck, knee, fingers, and other places on the body. Examples of commercially available, wearable vibrotactile aids include the single-channel Minifonator (Siemens Hearing Instruments); the single-channel Minivib 3 (AB Special Instruments, Sweden), the two-channel Tactaid II+ (Audiological Engineering Corporation), and the Tactaid 7, which is the most recent multi-channel tactile aid (Osberger, 1990).

The Tactaid 7, the most sophisticated device to date, has seven transducers in a vibrator array in a pouch worn over the sternum or rib areas to have contact with bone. There is also a processor package with an array of seven green lights corresponding to each vibrator. Different speech sounds stimulate each vibrator. The Tactaid 7 uses a place-of-stimulation code to convey different speech information.

Research has shown that children and adults who have little or no residual hearing benefit more from a tactile aid than they do from conventional hearing aids (Weisenberger & Miller, 1987). Nevertheless, the performance of even the highest functioning tactile-aid users does not equal the performance of multi-channel cochlear implant users (Osberger, Maso, & Sam, 1993; Tyler, Moore, & Kuk, 1989).

There is, however, some promising research using tactile aids with infants and preschool children with dual sensory impairments. Specifically, Franklin (1989), conducted a 3-year study of six students (aged 2 to 18 years) who had confirmed vision and hearing impairments. The children wore vibrotactile and electrotactile devices; results indicated that there was a positive effect on their communicative skills. For each child, three communicative behaviors were chosen, and communication was defined as "interaction with the environment." Children who wore the vibrotactile device demonstrated significantly more of the selected communicative behaviors than students who wore the electrotactile device. Use of either device increased targeted behaviors more than when no device was worn. Additionally, changes were observed in non-targeted behaviors. For example, one child began to lift her head in response to the vibrotactile stimulation; she had previously required physical stroking on her neck before lifting her head. Another child began to spontaneously vocalize *ah* and feel the electrovibrator for feedback.

Unfortunately, there are drawbacks to the use of vibrotactile or electrotactile devices. First, all persons who are fitted with a tactile aid require extensive training with the device to learn how to decode the vibratory patterns to understand speech; such training requires time and expertise (Osberger, 1990). If a vibrotactile device is recommended, a suggested training guide is the TARGO (Tactaid Reference Guide and Orientation), developed by Robbins, Hesketh, and Bivins and published in 1993 by Audiological Engineering (Somerville, MA). The TARGO has sequential levels of training: exposure, detection beginning pattern perception, advanced pattern perception, and segmental contrasts.

Second, the availability of tactile devices is limited. The cost of a Tactaid 7 is approximately $3000.

Third, the devices may be heavy for some small children, especially for a child with a motoric impairment such as cerebral palsy. Placement of the Tactaid also is a problem for children with motoric impairments; children with alternative means of ambulation (e.g., rolling, creeping) may have fewer options for the placement of the device. Certainly, further research is needed on training methods and use of vibrotactile devices.

Cochlear Implants

A cochlear implant is a surgically inserted biomedical device designed to provide sound information to children and adults who experience severe to profound hearing loss. The cochlear implant is **not** like a hearing aid. In fact, the implant bypasses some of the damaged parts of the inner ear; coded electrical signals stimulate different hearing nerve fibers which then send information to the brain (Clark, Cowan, & Dowell, 1997; Tyler, 1993).

Candidacy

As cochlear implant technology improves and as more outcome data are available, candidacy criteria are changing and becoming more liberal. General trends are that children are being implanted at an increasingly younger age and they have more hearing (Tucker, 1998). Why? Because data continue to show that the younger a child is when implanted, the better are the desired outcomes of meaningful spoken language and literacy development due to stimulation of critical auditory brain centers during the early years of neural plasticity (Estabrooks, 1998).

Following are general preoperative selection criteria for children. There might be some variability between implant centers—and it is the implant team that ultimately determines who is or is not a candidate.

- Ages 18 months and older.
- Severe to profound bilateral sensorineural hearing loss.
- Intact auditory nerve.
- Little benefit from hearing aids—although the term "benefit" is subject to interpretation.
- A 3- to 6-month trial with well-fitted hearing aids typically is recommended in conjunction with intensive auditory therapy. These criteria may be waived under certain circumstances, such as a history of meningitis with subsequent cochlear ossification.
- No medical contraindications to undergoing surgery.
- No active middle-ear disease.
- An educational setting that emphasizes auditory therapy and communication.
- The family and, if possible, the candidate should be highly motivated and have realistic expectations.

The following criteria often are added to the above in determining who to refer to an implant center for evaluation:

- A desired outcome for the child of spoken language and reading skills consistent with hearing peers.
- Mainstream classroom placement.

■ When wearing well-fitted hearing aids, the child is unable to understand speech at normal conversational levels without lipreading. The child can score up to 20% on open-set single syllable words and still be referred to an implant center. A child with a severe to profound hearing loss who demonstrates some benefit from hearing aids typically makes rapid and substantial progress with a cochlear implant. Why? Some benefit from hearing aids means that the auditory centers of the brain have been stimulated so that when the superior "keyboard" of the cochlear implant is provided, the child already has a neurological network in place for sound utilization.

■ Unaided thresholds of 90 dB or worse from 750 Hz through 8000 Hz.

■ An aided speech recognition threshold (the softest level that known speech material can just barely be recognized using a closed-set task) of 35 dB HL or worse. There is a distinction between hearing-aid gain and sound-quality benefit.

■ Aided distance hearing less than 10 ft for /s/ and less than 20 ft for *sh*. Distance hearing with an implant often can exceed 40 ft even for /s/.

Therefore, if a family previously was told (even in the recent past) that their child was not a candidate at that time—because he or she had too much residual hearing, or was getting too much gain from the hearing aid, had some open-set discrimination, or was too young or too old—they should ask the implant center for an updated opinion. Neither medicine nor technology is static. As we learn more about this wonderful device and about the possibilities it holds, different decisions will be made about candidacy.

Implant Description

Figure 5–17 depicts the components of the Mini System 22: a directional microphone, cable, and transmitter that is worn behind the ear; a speech processor that looks like a pocket calculator, weighs about 3.5 ounces, and is worn in a pocket or on a belt; and the actual cochlear implant which is the surgically implanted internal portion of the device—the magnet and receiver/stimulator are implanted in the mastoid process, and the banded array of 22 electrodes is implanted in the cochlea.

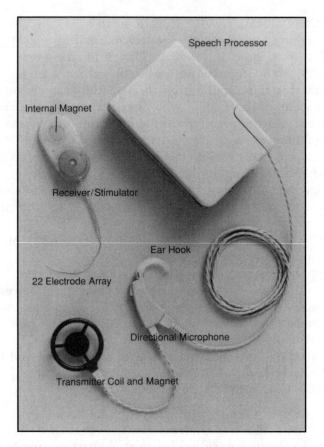

Figure 5–17. The components of the Mini System 22 Cochlear Implant. (Photo Courtesy of Cochlear Corporation)

Figure 5-18 depicts a schematic representation of the CLAR-ION Multi-Strategy cochlear implant electrode array.

Once implanted, the speech processor is custom programmed over several months for each child (see Figure 5–19). All current devices on the market have multiple program capacities that facilitate the mapping process and reduce the amount of time spent for mapping at the implant center. *Please note that if a child is not progressing as expected or behavior and performance alter in a negative direction, contact your implant center and check the integrity of the device's map/program first!*

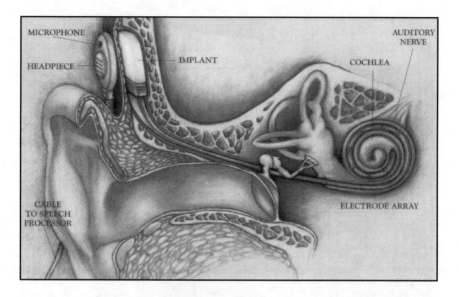

MICROPHONE

HEADPIECE

IMPLANT

AUDITORY NERVE

COCHLEA

CABLE TO SPEECH PROCESSOR

ELECTRODE ARRAY

Figure 5–18. Schematic representation of an electrode array in the cochlea. (From *Cochlear Implants for Infants and Children*, by J. G. Clark, R. S. C. Cowan, and R. C. Dowell, 1997, p. 510. San Diego, CA: Singular Publishing Group).

The Food and Drug Administration (FDA) approved the Nucleus 22-channel cochlear implant (Cochlear Corporation) for children in 1990; the Nucleus 24-channel cochlear implant was approved for children in June, 1998; the CLARION Multi-Strategy cochlear implant (Advanced Bionics Corporation) was approved for children in June, 1997; and the Austrian group Med-El, COMBIE 40+ cochlear implant, is now undergoing clinical trials in the United States. Improvements in design for all devices include increased battery life (from about 6 to about 16 hr); a telemetry system to help determine internal function of the device; troubleshooting signals (e.g., flashing lights, beeps, etc.) to notify parents and teachers if the head piece (magnet) falls off or the batteries are weakening; multiple program capacity; and sophisticated and rapid processing strategies that allow for improved speech perception (Tucker, 1998a). Ear-level speech processors also are becoming available (see Figure 5-20).

For more information about device design and benefit, please see Clark, Cowan, and Dowell (1997); Estabrooks (1998); and Tucker (1998a).

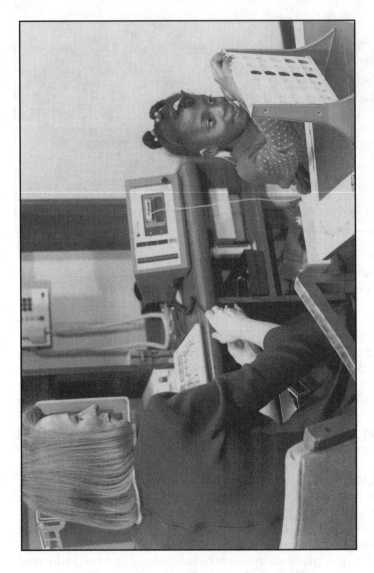

Figure 5–19. Once implanted and following a 4- to 6-week surgical recovery period, the speech processor is programmed. Programming occurs over several months, and the program may be modified as needed. The child above is indicating, by chips, whether she detects the sounds and if the sounds are comfortable. (Photo Courtesy of Cochlear Corporation)

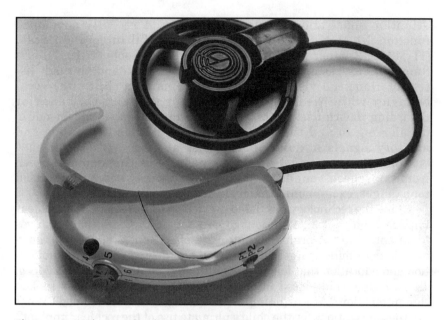

Figure 5–20. The "ear level" ESPrit™ speech processor in the Nucleus-24 system. (Source: *Cochlear Implants for Infants and Children: Advances,* by J. G. Clark, R. S. C. Cowan, and R. C. Dowell, 1997, p. 5. San Diego, CA: Singular Publishing Group).

Benefit

Data are very exciting and show that children with multichannel cochlear implants demonstrate significant improvements in all areas of speech perception compared with their preoperative performance with vibrotactile or conventional hearing aids (Miyamoto, Osberger, & Robbins, 1992; Sehgal, Kirk, Svirsky, Ertmer, & Osberger, 1998). Benefits range from improved detection of sounds to understanding speech without lipreading and include easy telephone use (Estabrooks, 1998; Sehgal, Kirk, Svirsky, & Miyamoto, 1998). In general, children who benefit the most from cochlear implantation are younger and/or received the implant after a shorter duration of deafness, are in good auditory-based training programs, and have families who are firmly committed to the training process. An additional key factor is the length of time the child uses the implant. Children who have used their device for more than 3 years are still showing substantial improvement.

Assessing cochlear implant benefit (as well as hearing aid and FM benefit) in infants and young children has been challenging because this population has limited communication skills, limited attention span, and immature behaviors. A recently developed functional tool, the Infant-Toddler Meaningful Integration Scale (IT-MAIS; Zimmerman-Phillips, Osberger, & Robbins, 1997), is a functional assessment that describes, over time and through listening alone (no visual cues), such items as a child's (a) vocal behavior while wearing hearing aid or implant, (b) behavior regarding device use, (c) response to name in quiet and in noise, (d) alerting to and then recognizing environmental sounds and auditory signals in quiet and in noise at home and then in new environments without being prompted, (e) distinguishing speech from nonspeech sounds, and (f) spontaneously associating vocal tone (anger, excitement, anxiety) with its meaning.

Like the technology discussed previously in this chapter, a cochlear implant is only a tool; analogous to a computer keyboard that improves "data entry" to the brain. The ultimate effectiveness of the tool, however, is determined largely by the type and degree of aural rehabilitation and education that follow implantation (Boothroyd, Geers, & Moog, 1991). Is the child placed in an environment that emphasizes spoken communication? Are listening skills systematically developed? What are the expectations for the child's ultimate use of the cochlear implant?

Data entry and auditory-linguistic skill building take time, often years. The child who has an implant needs to be taught to interpret and derive meaning from the sounds that now enter his or her brain via the cochlear implant. The child who has access to an appropriate, auditory-based program has the best opportunity to benefit from a cochlear implant.

It seems logical that if a new "keyboard" is to be provided for a child who has not previously had a keyboard, all efforts should be geared toward helping the child learn how to use the newly entered data.

■ SUMMARIES OF AMPLIFICATION TECHNOLOGIES

Appendixes 5A through 5D summarize the information in this chapter by presenting fact sheets that describe construction, use, responsibilities and tips about hearing aids (Appendix 5A); personal FM systems (Appendix 5B); sound-field FM systems (Appendix 5C); and a mild gain hard-wired system (Appendix 5D). A how-to guide for use of a hard-wired mild gain amplifier with remote microphone is provided in Appendix 5E, and a protocol for pediatric hearing and amplification management is provided in Appendix 5F.

Other assistive listening devices are available, such as infrared and loop systems (Compton, 1993). The hearing technologies selected for discussion are most appropriate for the population addressed in this book.

■ APPENDIX 5A. SUMMARY OF HEARING AIDS

A. Description

1. Hearing aids are like miniature public address systems that are worn by the individual user.

2. Hearing aids do not correct the hearing impairment or "fix" the person's ear. Rather, hearing aids alter the acoustic input from the environment by making sounds louder and by shaping them to make them accessible to the ear with a hearing impairment. Shaping means that if a person has more impairment for high frequencies or pitches, more amplification is provided for high frequencies than for the mid or low pitches. On the other hand, if a person has more hearing impairment in the low frequencies, more power is provided for those frequencies.

3. Hearing aids typically are the first amplification devices employed when a person is found to have a hearing impairment. However, because hearing aids function best in a quiet environment when the talker is very close to the listener, additional hearing technologies are needed to access diverse listening environments (e.g., classrooms, cars, outdoors). *In fact, a hearing aid might not be the first choice for amplification; a personal FM unit might be fitted before or instead of a hearing aid.*

4. Hearing aids for children must be fitted by an audiologist, and the hearing aid must be worn by the child for whom it was fitted.

5. Once infants or children have been provided access to the auditory environment and to spoken communication, they then can be taught the meaning of incoming sounds. Thus, hearing aids are the first step in the learning process; they facilitate the *reception* of sounds.

B. Parts of a Hearing Aid

Regardless of style, all hearing aids have the following components:

1. Microphone—receives the acoustic signal (sounds from the environment) and changes the sounds into an electric signal.

2. Amplifying Circuit—shapes the sound, now in the form of an electric current, and makes it louder.

3. Battery—provides power for the hearing aid.

4. Receiver—changes the amplified and shaped electrical signal back into an acoustic signal (sound) that can be heard. A receiver is a microphone in reverse.

5. Earmold—connected to a hearing aid—fits in the ear to hold the hearing aid in place and to deliver the newly amplified and shaped sound to the ear of the wearer. The earmold is

an important part of a hearing aid. For a child, the ear-mold must be made of soft material and fit comfortably and snugly. It also must be appropriately acoustically tuned. For example, earmolds with flared bores (wide openings) amplify best the higher pitches necessary to hear consonant sounds such as p, sh, s, and th.

C. **Styles of Hearing Aids**
   1. Behind-the-ear (BTE) or ear-level or over-the-ear hearing aids. This style fits comfortably and snugly behind the ear with tubing and earmold connecting the hearing aid to the ear. This is the most appropriate style of hearing aid for children.
   2. Body style hearing aid. The microphone, amplifying circuit, and battery are located in a small case that is worn on the body in a pouch or harness, with a connecting wire to a button receiver that snaps into the earmold. Body-type hearing aids used to be the most common style for children because they provided the most power and because they could be secured to the child. However, body-style hearing aids rarely are used today because ear-level hearing aids can provide enough power for even profound hearing impairments, and because the microphone location of the ear-level hearing aid (on the ear) is superior acoustically to a microphone location on the body.
   3. In-the-ear (ITE) hearing aids. All hearing aid components are built into the earmold which fits in the ear. Although in-the-ear hearing aids are popular with adults, they are rarely appropriate for children because
      a. A child's ear grows and thus the hearing aid needs to be changed, sometimes every few months (an adult's ear does not grow).
      b. In-the-ear hearing aids rarely have the flexible tone, output, and telecoil adjustments needed for children.
      c. In-the-ear hearing aids are not powerful enough for severe-to-profound hearing impairments and they often feedback (squeal) on children regardless of degree of hearing impairment.
      d. In-the-ear hearing aids are built into hard earmolds that, if broken, can cut and damage the child's ear. Children must have SOFT earmolds to protect them and to allow an appropriate fit.
      e. In-the-ear hearing aids cannot be coupled easily to the assistive listening devices that must be used in various learning domains.

    f. In-the-ear hearing aids are difficult to secure in the soft and small ear of a child so they fall out and are lost or damaged more often than ear-level hearing aids.

4. In-the-canal (ITC) and completely-in-the-canal (CIC) hearing aids: They are similar to in-the-ear aids, but smaller; the entire hearing aid fits deeper in the ear canal. The instrument is only slightly visible. Relative to fitting hearing aids on children, the same difficulties apply to canal-style hearing aids as apply to in-the-ear hearing aids, only more so!

D. Questions to Ask the Audiologist About Hearing Aids Worn by Children

1. Which specific speech sounds can the child hear while wearing the hearing aids? Ask for aided and unaided audiograms with a written comparison of aided and unaided sensitivity for speech sounds that are spoken at an average conversational level of loudness (45 dB HL).

2. If the child has a hearing impairment in both ears, two hearing aids should be worn unless a monaural fitting (only one hearing aid) has proven to be superior. If the child has only one hearing aid, ask the audiologist why.

3. The most suitable hearing aids for children typically are ear-level hearing aids with flexible internal controls that can change the amplifying characteristics of the hearing aid and strong telecoils with direct input to allow coupling to an FM unit. In addition, the external settings on the hearing aid should include a volume control wheel and switches: M (to turn on the hearing aid microphone), T (to activate the telecoil), and MT (to turn on the microphone and telecoil at the same time). Ask the audiologist to show you all of the settings, wheels, and switches on the hearing aid, explain their use to you, and show you where all of the switches and volume control wheel should be positioned. If the child's hearing aid does not have all of the above-mentioned features, ask why.

4. Take a close look at the child's earmold(s). It should be made of a soft, clear, hypoallergenic material and be clean and free of ear wax. A clear earmold rather than a tinted one is suggested because some persons have allergic skin reactions to the pigments used in tinted earmolds. Clear earmolds and tubing are visually more pleasing. Earmolds should be removed from the hearing aid and washed, at least weekly (children who have a tendency to get ear canal

infections should have their earmolds washed daily) with a mild detergent. They should be dried thoroughly inside and out with an air blower before being replaced on the hearing aid. Do not use heat to dry the earmold. Ask your audiologist whether the earmolds have been acoustically modified, and if not, whether earmold modifications could facilitate reception of speech sounds. In addition, if the child has had ventilating tubes surgically inserted in the eardrums for medical reasons, vents (holes) in the earmolds might be necessary to allow air into the ear canal. If you have any questions about how or why certain earmold designs were selected, do not hesitate to ask the audiologist. Note that new earmolds may be needed every few months for a baby or very young child because of ear growth.

5. Ask the audiologist to *demonstrate* hearing aid checking and troubleshooting techniques. Family counseling and training about hearing aid care is critical. A dead hearing aid is worse than nothing at all because the earmold then acts like an earplug. Over 50% of hearing aids malfunction on any given day. *When a child wears a hearing aid, his or her "ear" begins at the microphone of the hearing aid.* The only way to know if the hearing aid is working, is to **listen to it**—at least once a day before beginning school. You will need a hearing aid stethoscope, a battery tester, and air blower (to clean moisture out of the earmold), an earwax remover (to remove earwax from the earmold), and extra batteries. Ask the school audiologist to provide an inservice to allow you to practice with these tools. Also ask how to use the Ling 6 Sound Test to perform a listening check. The Ling 6 Sounds are ah, ee, oo, sh, s, and m; these sounds were selected because they contain speech energy that is representative of all English speech sounds.

6. Ask about how long the batteries should function: battery life. Hearing aid batteries may last from a few days to a few weeks depending on the power requirements of the hearing aid and on how long and often the hearing aid is worn. Most hearing aid malfunctions can be traced to the battery. Therefore, the first thing to try, if the hearing aid is not working or not working appropriately, is to test and change the battery.

7. Ask the audiologist about managing moisture in the hearing aid. Especially in humid environments and for individuals who perspire, moisture can be a real problem. The hearing

aid can stop working until the moisture is dried out. Over time, constant moisture can cause erosion that results in costly repair. When not worn, hearing aids should be kept in a container with moisture-absorbing material. Teachers or therapists might want to have extra moisture-absorbing containers at school so the hearing aids can be placed in them during nap time.

8. Because a hearing aid is effective only when the speaker is close to the user and the environment is quiet, ask the audiologist which assistive listening devices would be most appropriate in various learning environments (e.g., personal FM unit, sound-field FM, or a hard-wired unit for individual instruction). Often, assistive listening devices are fitted at the same time as the hearing aid, and most certainly, the hearing aids must be able to couple to assistive listening devices.

9. Ask the audiologist how often electroacoustic analyses of the hearing aids should be performed. A listening check should be performed at least once a day, but a thorough electroacoustic analysis of the hearing aid's output, frequency response, and distortion typically is done every 3 months for infants and very young children. Remember, the hearing aid is the device that allows the child to receive acoustic information from the environment. If the hearing aid is not working appropriately, valuable intervention time is lost, learning is sabotaged, and brain development is compromised.

10. Ask the audiologist whether probe-microphone real-ear measurements have been performed to determine the aided frequency response and amplified signal intensity in the child's ear canal.

11. Ask the audiologist if a multiple-memory hearing aid, a remote control device, or advanced signal processing would be useful enough for your child to warrant the considerable additional expense. Could a more conventional flexible hearing aid achieve the same target amplification objectives? Remember, an FM system with its accompanying remote microphone ALWAYS will be necessary to facilitate over-hearing and distance learning in a classroom learning situation and at home.

E. Who Might Benefit from a Hearing Aid?

1. Normal hearing sensitivity for a child is *15 dB HL or better* at all frequencies and no air-bone gap. No air-bone gap means that the middle ears are normal.

2. Remember, hearing impairment is not an either/or issue. Even a slight hearing impairment can interfere with the reception of intelligible speech.

3. Babies of any age can have their hearing tested.

4. The point is, any time a permanent hearing impairment is identified, even a minimal hearing impairment, the baby or child is a candidate for hearing aids. Even infants in the first 3 months of life can be fitted with hearing aids.

5. There are some instances (e.g., when a child has a fluctuating hearing impairment, a unilateral hearing impairment, or a mild permanent hearing impairment) when it may be more effective to fit a mild gain personal FM unit or a sound-field system instead of, or before, a personal hearing aid. A child with one of the hearing impairments just listed may do fine in a quiet, one-to-one learning situation, but the child **will** have difficulty in a typical, noisy, distracting learning environment such as a classroom. We now know that preferential seating is not an effective way of overcoming the negative effects of distance and noise on the speech signal (Leavitt & Flexer, 1991).

6. If speech is being used as the means of communication, instruction, or intervention, there is **no** instance where hearing does not matter. Unless the instructor is able to serve as the amplifier by speaking in a full, clear voice into the ear of the child at all times, some form of amplification technology will be necessary. *No hearing impairment is insignificant, no age is too young, and no disability is too severe to consider the use of amplification.*

F. **What Are the Child's Responsibilities for Managing the Hearing Aid?**

1. The level of responsibility of the child is determined by the child's age and ability.

2. The expectation is that the child will be able to participate to some degree in the use and maintenance of the hearing aid.

3. With appropriate intervention, by the time a typical child is in kindergarten, he or she should be able to insert and remove the earmold and hearing aid, notify parents or teachers when the hearing aid is malfunctioning, adjust the volume control to accommodate to different acoustic environments, and test and change batteries.

4. The levels of responsibility for a child's hearing aid management include:

a. Keeping the hearing aid on. Some children wear the hearing aid during all waking hours within 24 hours of fitting. Others require up to 1 month to adapt to the mechanical feel of the earmold and to the changes in their acoustic environment caused by hearing amplified sound. Once the audiologist has determined that the earmold fits well and that the amplification is appropriate, the child should be wearing the hearing aids during all waking hours within 1 month of the fitting. If the child refuses to wear the hearing aids, work with the audiologist to rule out: outer or middle ear infection (which may require a medical consultation); pain or discomfort caused by the earmold; inappropriate amplification (too loud, too soft, wrong shaping of the sound); malfunctioning hearing aid (the hearing aid may be shorting-out, have static, or may not work at all); or a change in the child's hearing status (hearing may have worsened or improved).

b. Indicate in some way to parents or teachers that the hearing aid is malfunctioning. Begin with simply knowing when the hearing aid is on or off. Then progress to having the child determine intermittent or inappropriate function. Hearing aids do break, and batteries do go dead. If a listening check is performed by parents and teachers only once a day, and if the child cannot notify them when the hearing aid is off or malfunctioning in between checks, then valuable learning time is lost and brain development is compromised.

c. Insert the earmold and hearing aid. Initially, the baby or child should be taught to not touch the hearing aid at all to avoid damage or loss due to the child removing and dropping, chewing on, or losing the hearing aid. As the child matures, the child might learn to remove the hearing aid with supervision. Inserting the earmold is more difficult than removing it because insertion requires more complex motor control.

d. Regulating the volume of the hearing aid. Different acoustic environments require more or less amplification. Initially, the child can be taught to ask for more or less power (some indication that sounds are too loud or too soft). As the child matures, the child should have independent control of the volume. Hearing aid volume wheels are quite small and often tricky to operate. Hearing aids can be special-ordered with raised volume controls and, in some cases, with a remote control volume adjustor.

e. Checking and changing the battery. Because batteries do not last long in hearing aids and because the most frequent source of hearing aid malfunction is related to batteries, control of the batteries is very important. Unfortunately, batteries are poisonous if put in the nose, mouth, or swallowed, so teaching battery care to a child requires careful supervision. Initially, to protect the baby or child, hearing aids can be ordered with tamper-resistant battery compartments. As the child matures, he or she can be taught to check the charge of the battery by using a battery checker, typically a volt meter. Then, the child can be taught to appropriately place the battery in the battery compartment of the hearing aid.

f. Basic hearing aid maintenance. As the child develops maturity and motor skills, he or she can be responsible for keeping the earmold free of ear wax and for washing it. In addition, every time the child removes the hearing aid, it should be placed safely in the container with moisture-absorbing material. The child also can learn to notify parents when new batteries need to be purchased.

g. Basic hearing aid trouble-shooting skills. If the hearing aid is not working at all, working intermittently, or squealing, the child can be taught some simple techniques to locate the source of the problem. Ask the audiologist to work with you in designing a program to teach the child to check the battery, earmold, tubing, hearing aid case, and so forth to see if the problem can be identified.

h. Decisions for use of different types of amplification devices. Because different listening environments demand different types of amplification technologies, an older child can be taught to determine the use of appropriate devices. For example, the child might turn on his or her FM unit in the classroom or use a telephone amplifier when speaking on the telephone.

i. Ask the audiologist for assistance in progressing through all of the levels of hearing aid responsibility listed above.

Maximum independence and control, to the fullest extent possible, is the goal for children who use amplification technology.

■ APPENDIX 5B. SUMMARY OF PERSONAL FM UNITS

A. Description

1. FM stands for frequency-modulated radio transmission. FM means that the signal is frequency modulated onto a carrier wave that is sent from the transmitter to the receiver where it is demodulated and delivered to the listener.

2. An FM unit is an assistive listening device that improves the speech-to-noise (S/N) ratio by use of a *remote microphone* that can be placed close to the sound source. The more favorable the S/N ratio, the more intelligible the speech signal received by the child. Because sound is degraded as it travels across a distance from the source to the listener, the closer the listener is to the speaker, either physically or technologically, the better access the listener will have to a clear speech signal.

3. Any time a child with a hearing problem is in a classroom setting, an FM unit will be necessary to provide an improved S/N ratio to enhance the intelligibility of the teacher's speech. A hearing aid alone is never enough in a classroom setting or any time the speaker cannot be close to the child.

4. A personal FM unit is like having your own tiny private radio station that transmits and receives on a single frequency.

5. There are no wires connecting speaker and listener allowing free mobility for both parties. The transmission range is about 200 feet or more.

6. The parent, teacher, clinician, or peer wears the small transmitter microphone clipped on a collar or no farther away than 6 inches from the speaker's mouth. The microphone also can be placed close to the speakers of a television, video monitor, stereo, or computer.

7. Think of the FM microphone as the child's "third" ear and put that third ear within 6 inches of whatever you want the child to hear. You do not have to physically move the child close to each relevant sound source. Simply move the microphone transmitter.

8. The FM receiver is worn by the child and must be set to the same radio frequency as the microphone/transmitter for the child to receive the desired radio signal.

B. Features of FM Systems

1. FM systems can be quite complicated to fit appropriately to a child because of the numerous setting and fitting options that are available. Consequently, many decisions must be

made. *An audiologist must be involved in clinic and class-room evaluations of FM settings and function.*

2. Many models of FM units are available with multiple options for internal and external settings. The audiologist will decide which FM unit and which coupling arrangement to use based on:

   a. The listening needs of the child.

   b. The demands of the listening environments.

   c. The flexibility of the child's hearing aid. Hopefully, the child's hearing aid will have many features that will allow it to receive signals from an FM unit.

   d. No single coupling arrangement is automatically supe-rior for all children, because there are many child, FM, environment, and hearing aid variables.

3. An FM unit may be fitted instead of a hearing aid. The FM receiver can send the signal directly to the listener's ear through one of several options:

   a. Use of an earpiece that is connected from the FM receiver to the listener's ear by a wire.

   b. Use of Walkman-type monophonic (not stereo) head-phones that are connected from the FM receiver to the listener's ear by a wire.

   c. Use of a button-type external receiver that snaps into a cus-tom-made earmold that fits into the child's ear. There is a wire connecting the FM receiver to the external button receiver.

   d. Some FM receivers are designed to function as hearing aids as well as radio receivers. The child takes off his or her hearing aid when wearing this type of FM system because the FM receiver serves as both the hearing aid and FM radio receiver.

   e. Recent new technological developments have provided the option of a hearing aid and FM receiver both housed together in a behind-the-ear hearing aid case; there is no body-worn FM receiver. The child can, by moving a switch, have the unit function as a hearing aid only, an FM receiver only, or as both a hearing aid and FM receiver at the same time.

4. The typical FM receiver may be coupled to the child's personal hearing aids through one of the following options; that is, the signal from the FM receiver is fed to the child's ear *through* the child's hearing aids:

   a. The signal from the FM receiver is sent to a wire or loop that is attached to the FM receiver and is worn around the child's neck. The neckloop generates a magnetic field that is picked up by the T attachment on the child's hearing aid (provided, of course, that the child's hearing aid is equipped with an appropriate T or telephone coil). There are no wires connecting the neckloop with the hearing aid, and the neckloop can be worn under clothing.

  b. The signal from the FM receiver can be sent via a direct input cord that attaches from the FM receiver to the child's hearing aid. The hearing aid must be equipped with a special "direct input" feature.

Each attachment option can change the power output and frequency response of the equipment. *An audiologist must be involved in the initial setting of the equipment and in any subsequent coupling or setting changes.*

C. **Questions to Ask the Audiologist About FM Units Worn by Children in Your Program**

1. Which specific speech sounds can the child hear while wearing the FM unit? Ask for a written comparison of unaided, aided, and FM sensitivity for speech sounds spoken at an average conversational level of loudness. Keep in mind that the hearing aid microphone is always on the child, whereas the FM microphone is always (or should be) close to the desired sound source. Thus, the remote microphone of the FM unit, if appropriately fitted, will always have an advantage over the microphone of the hearing aid because it can be closer to the desired signal.

2. Can the equipment be set so that the child can hear the teacher (through the FM microphone) and classmates (through the hearing aid microphone) at the same time? Are the settings flexible enough to allow the child to hear only the teacher (FM microphone), or only the classmates/environment (hearing aid microphone)?

3. Where should all of the controls be positioned on the FM unit and on the hearing aid when the FM unit is coupled to the hearing aid? **If the hearing aid and FM unit controls are not in the proper position, the child may not receive any signal at all!**

4. Ask the audiologist to *demonstrate* FM checking and trouble-shooting techniques. Over 50% of amplification devices are not working at any given time. The only way to know for sure whether the FM unit is transmitting and receiving appropriately is to *listen to it in the environment in which it is used* at least once a day. The FM unit might be free from interference in the school office, but pick up computer

noise in another room of the same building. Note that radio signals from modular telephones and pagers also might be picked up by an FM unit if they are on the same radio frequency. You will need a hearing aid stethoscope to listen to the receiver if an earmold is being used. Ask the audiologist to provide an inservice to allow you to practice checking the device. Earmold issues and care are covered in the fact sheet on hearing aids.

5. Ask about battery life and charging batteries. Some FM rechargeable batteries may not retain their charge for even 1 full day. As the battery weakens, the FM transmission range decreases and interference, static, and buzzing occur.

6. Ask about modifications of equipment settings or use if you want the child to be able to hear his or her own voice as well as the voice of the teacher or parent.

7. If you will be using several FM units in the same building, ask the audiologist about coordinating transmission frequencies to avoid interference.

8. Ask about home, car, and community use of the FM system to expand distance and incidental listening and learning. When would the FM be appropriate and how could it be used most efficiently?

D. Who Can Benefit From an FM Unit?

1. Any time a child with a hearing problem is in a classroom or cannot be close to the speaker, an improved S/N ratio is necessary to facilitate the reception of clear speech.

2. Children who wear hearing aids can have the FM unit coupled to their hearing aids, **if** their hearing aids have the appropriate features. But hearing aids alone will not substitute for an FM unit in a classroom or in any environment where the speaker cannot be consistently close to the listener. It used to be thought that preferential seating was sufficient. However, recent information about classroom acoustics and the speech signal show that access to a clear and consistent speech signal is not possible in a typical learning environment.

3. There are some instances (e.g., when a child has a fluctuating hearing impairment, a unilateral hearing impairment, or a slight permanent hearing impairment) when it may be more effective to fit a mild-gain personal FM unit or a sound-field system instead of, or before, a personal hearing aid. A child with the types of hearing impairments just listed might do fine in a quiet, one-to-one learning situation,

but the same child *will* have difficulty in a typical, noisy, distracting classroom. It should be noted that a personal FM system is not the same as a sound-field FM system. The two systems are not interchangeable; different decisions govern the recommendation of each.

E. What Are the Child's Responsibilities for the FM Unit?

1. The level of responsibility of the child is dependent on the child's age and ability.
2. The expectation is that the child will be able to participate in some way in the use and maintenance of the FM unit.
3. With appropriate intervention, by the time a typical child is in kindergarten, he or she should be able to understand and use an FM unit.
4. The levels of responsibility for FM use include:
   a. See the Hearing Aid Summary Sheet (Appendix 5A) for more details because FM use and hearing aid use may be tied together.
   b. Keep the FM unit on. If an FM unit is being used to supplement hearing aid function, the child may need to first adjust to the hearing aid before adjusting to the feel and sound of the FM unit.
   c. Indicate in some way to parents or teachers when the FM unit is malfunctioning. Begin by simply knowing when the FM unit is on or off. Then progress to having the child determine intermittent or inappropriate function. Note that someone with normal hearing also needs to perform listening checks on the equipment. The child who has a hearing impairment cannot be responsible totally for determining FM function.
   d. Regulate the volume of the FM unit. It is unrealistic to assume that a single volume setting will be appropriate for all sound sources. Ideally, a child can decide whether a soft spoken teacher needs more FM volume, whereas a louder video system necessitates that the FM volume be reduced.
   e. Put the FM unit in the battery charger at the end of each day of use.
   f. Basic FM maintenance and trouble-shooting skills.
   g. Decisions for use of different amplification technologies. The child ultimately may be able to decide when to switch his or her equipment settings from using the hearing aid only, to using the FM only, or to using the FM and hearing aids together at the same time.

■ APPENDIX 5C. SOUND-FIELD FM SYSTEMS

A. Description

1. FM stands for frequency-modulated radio transmission. The signal is frequency modulated onto a carrier wave that is sent from the transmitter to the receiver where it is demodulated and delivered to the listener.

2. A sound-field FM system is one type of assistive listening device that improves the speech-to-noise (S/N) ratio by the use of a *remote microphone* that can be placed close to the desired sound source. The more favorable the S/N ratio, the clearer and more intelligible the speech signal received by the child.

3. Sound-field FM technology offers a way to amplify an entire classroom (or therapy room, or room in the home) through the use of two, three, or four wall- or ceiling-mounted loudspeakers. Sound-field systems are like high fidelity, wireless, public address systems.

4. The parent, clinician, or teacher wears a wireless FM microphone transmitter, just like the one worn for a personal FM unit, and the radio signal is sent to an amplifier that is connected to the loudspeakers. There are no wires connecting the teacher with the equipment, which allows the teacher to move about freely.

5. All of the children in the classroom benefit from an improved and consistent S/N ratio no matter where they or the teacher are located.

6. Thus, sound-field FM simply increases the loudness of speech relative to background noise throughout the room or classroom.

B. Features of Sound-field FM Systems

1. A major difference between a personal FM unit and a sound-field (classroom) FM system is that the personal FM can provide an extremely favorable S/N ratio (about +20 to +30 dB), whereas the sound-field FM can provide a S/N ratio of only about +10 to +15 dB. A S/N of +10 dB may not be sufficient for children with more severe hearing impairments or for those who have great difficulty focusing their attention. A typical, quiet classroom has an inconsistent S/N of only +4 dB, so sound-field FM certainly is beneficial for many children.

2. As discussed above, sound-field FM is not a replacement for personal FM systems. One possible arrangement would be to amplify the entire classroom via sound-field FM equip-

ment, which would benefit children with normal hearing or mild fluctuating hearing impairments. Children in the classroom who wear hearing aids and have more severe hearing impairments could wear personal FM receivers tuned to the same frequency as the sound-field system so that the teacher need wear only a single, wireless microphone transmitter.

3. A sound-field FM system may be recommended instead of a personal hearing aid for children with mild, fluctuating hearing impairments or unilateral hearing impairments.
4. Because sound-field systems benefit the entire classroom (all children hear the amplified sound), the equipment does not call attention to children who might particularly need the amplification. The wearer of a personal FM receiver is obvious, the "needy" listener of sound-field amplification is not.
5. The function of a sound-field FM unit is much easier to trouble-shoot than is the function of hearing aids or personal FM units. *Everyone* hears the sound-field FM; only the wearer of the hearing aids or personal FM hears the sound coming through those units. Interference, feedback, static, or distortion are immediately obvious to all who hear a sound-field FM unit.
6. Cellular telephones and pagers can cause acoustic interference if they are on the same radio frequency as the sound-field, or any FM, equipment.
7. Sound-field FM is most effective for group instruction.
8. Individual or small group instruction also can be orchestrated with sound-field equipment.
9. The teacher can allow students to talk into the microphone when they are addressing the class, such as for "show and tell."
10. A personal sound-field FM unit can fit on a child's desk and can be carried from class to class easily.

C. **Questions to Ask the Audiologist About Sound-field FM Systems**
   1. Where should the loudspeakers be positioned to allow the most even and consistent improvement in S/N ratio throughout the classroom? Improper positioning can amplify classroom reverberation thereby interfering with speech intelligibility.
   2. How much S/N ratio improvement has been obtained in the particular classroom in question? What does this S/N ratio improvement mean relative to hearing the teacher's speech?

3. Ask the audiologist to demonstrate sound-field FM use and trouble-shooting techniques. Note that the primary cause of static and distortion is a weak battery in the teacher's microphone/transmitter.

4. Ask the audiologist to demonstrate how the equipment might be modified for small group instruction. For example, how would some of the loudspeakers be disconnected?

5. If several sound-field FM units are in use in the same building, all must be on different radio frequencies to avoid "cross-talk." Thus, the frequencies of all FM units, personal and sound-field, must be coordinated throughout a building, or chaos could result.

6. Ask the audiologist whether the sound-field unit is providing enough amplification for all of the children in your classroom. Might some children also need hearing aids and/or personal FM units?

D. Who Might Benefit From Sound-field (Classroom) Amplification?

1. Children with normal hearing can benefit from sound-field FM because the improved S/N ratio creates a more favorable learning environment. If children can hear better, they have an opportunity to learn more efficiently.

2. Children with fluctuating conductive hearing impairments (primarily caused by ear infections or ear wax) can benefit.

3. Children with unilateral hearing impairments (hearing impairment in one ear; the other ear is normal) also will benefit from classroom amplification.

4. Children with slight permanent hearing impairments might benefit more from sound-field FM than from a hearing aid.

5. Children with mild-to-moderate hearing impairments who wear hearing aids might do as well with sound-field FM as they would with a personal FM system. Consult with the audiologist to determine the appropriate S/N ratio enhancing equipment for this population.

6. Children with normal hearing who have difficulty "processing" or understanding speech might benefit from sound-field FM. As previously stated, a child with central auditory processing difficulties might need the more favorable S/N ratio provided by a personal FM unit. Discuss FM technology with the audiologist.

7. Children for whom English is a second language benefit from the increased signal redundancy provided by a sound-field FM.

8. Children with cochlear implants also require an improved S/N ratio due to distance from the teacher and background noise.
9. Teachers benefit from sound-field FM use due to decreased vocal abuse and strain.

E. What Are the Child's Responsibilities for the Sound-field Unit?

1. The child has no direct responsibility for the equipment because the equipment is not worn by the child.
2. The child could be taught to indicate in some way whether the amplified sound is too loud, too soft, or not clear enough.

■ APPENDIX 5D. SUMMARY OF MILD GAIN HARD-WIRED UNIT

A. Description

1. "Mild gain" means low power output. There are more powerful hard-wired units too, such as the William Sound PockeTalker.
2. "Hard-wired" means that the speaker and listener are connected by wires; there is no radio transmission.
3. There are many mild gain hard-wired devices on the market. The mild gain hard-wired unit referred to here is a small, inexpensive, portable, low power device.

B. Features of the Mild Gain Hard-wired Unit

1. This unit is comprised of inexpensive component parts obtained from Radio Shack. It has a small battery-operated miniamplifier, a small tie clip microphone, and Walkman type monophonic (as compared to stereophonic) earphones.
2. Note that the unit discussed here has an external microphone attached to the miniamplifier by a wire. The microphone is *not* built into the unit. The value of this unit is in the external (remote) microphone that can be moved close to the sound source thereby improving the Signal-to-Noise (S/N) ratio. A unit with a built-in microphone is **not** the same thing as discussed here; do not use a unit with a built-in microphone because you will not get an improvement in speech intelligibility.
3. This system is lightweight, portable, and costs about $50.00.
4. Up to four microphones can be used by inserting a series of three Y-adapters into the input jack of the miniamplifier. The number of headsets also can be expanded by using Y-adapters in the output jack of the miniamplifier. Whenever microphones or headsets are added, power output is reduced, and volume may need to be increased. Check with the audiologist.
5. Because this unit has the limitation of restricted mobility caused by the connecting wires between the microphone, miniamplifier and the headset, it is **not** suitable for classroom instruction.
6. *This unit works best in the restricted context of one-on-one instruction or in very small groups using Y-adapters; it is not intended to replace personal FM systems or hearing aids.*
7. The amplification provided by this hard-wired unit and remote microphone improves the S/N ratio, thereby focusing the child's attention on the desired auditory input.

8. The microphone can be moved back and forth from the teacher to the child to facilitate turn-taking.
9. The microphone is placed within 6 inches of the relevant sound source.
10. Always listen to the unit before you use it to make sure that it is functioning appropriately and stabilize the volume control (with a piece of tape) at the desired setting. The power output may be too loud if the volume is turned full-on and someone shouts into the microphone.

C. **Questions to Ask the Audiologist About the Hard-wired Unit**
1. How do you assemble the components (not at all difficult to do), and how do you insert the Y-adapters? How would you operate the unit off wall current rather than batteries?
2. If the child has a hearing impairment, is the unit providing enough amplification? That is, is the unit appropriate for a given child? Where should the volume be set?
3. How do you trouble-shoot the unit? Because there is no radio transmission, there is no radio interference with the unit. However, there can be static and distortion or electrical interference. Check the battery at the first sign of trouble.

D. **Who Can Benefit From Using a Hard-wired Unit?**
1. Populations that might benefit include:
   a. Children with normal hearing who have trouble focusing on auditory input or are easily distracted during individual instruction. Remember, this unit is **not** for group or classroom instruction.
   b. Children who have fluctuating hearing impairments caused primarily by ear infections or ear wax.
   c. Children with unilateral hearing impairments.
   d. Children with mild permanent hearing impairments.
2. Children who use a personal FM unit in the classroom can also use that unit during individual therapy or instruction; they would not need a hard-wired unit.
3. Children who use sound-field FM amplification for classroom instruction could benefit from the use of the hard-wired unit during individual therapy or instruction.
4. This unit can be purchased by families and used at home during reading and homework times.

E. **What Are the Child's Responsibilities for the Hard-wired Unit?**
1. The level of responsibility of the child is determined by the child's age and ability.

2. The expectation is that the child will be able to participate in some way in the use and maintenance of the equipment.
3. The levels of responsibility include:
   a. Keeping the Walkman earphones on his or her ears.
   b. Indicating in some way when the unit is malfunctioning.
   c. Regulating the volume of the hard-wired unit. Until the child can indicate his or her comfort level, the teacher sets the volume at the setting recommended by the audiologist (usually at a comfortable listening level for a person with normal hearing).
   d. Taking the unit out prior to instruction and putting it away at completion.

■ APPENDIX 5E. A HOW-TO GUIDE FOR USE OF A HARD-WIRED MILD GAIN AMPLIFIER WITH REMOTE MICROPHONE[1]

1. The audiologist and other members of the early intervention team begin by working together to establish dependent measures consistent with the goals and objectives of therapy for the child. These measures should be sensitive to language, speech, and behavioral goals that will demonstrate the effect of the assistive listening device on the child's performance. Examples of dependent measures are accuracy of the child's production of individual phonemes, duration of attention to the therapy activity, number of clinician prompts needed to facilitate the child's attention to task, and so on.

2. Demonstrate and practice the assembly of component parts, showing the use of the mini-phone jack adapter for multiple microphones or headsets.

3. If the parent, clinician, or teacher has normal hearing sensitivity, have the clinician set the gain of the unit to a comfortable listening level and do a listening check of the fidelity. The Ling Six Sound Test can be used: ah, oo, ee, sh, s, and m. The clinician must perform a listening check, holding the microphone approximately 6 inches from his or her mouth, every time the equipment is used. Then, if the child can respond, put the headset on the child and ask whether the volume is appropriate. If the child wishes the volume turned up or down, the clinician needs to listen to the unit again at the child-determined volume setting. Note that a child who is experiencing otitis media might want the gain increased. Stabilize the volume control, perhaps with a piece of tape.

4. Position the microphone no further than 6 inches from the mouth of the speaker. *Correct microphone positioning is critical for improvement of the speech-to-noise (S/N) ratio*, and the primary purpose of using this unit is to enhance the S/N ratio. Inappro-

---

[1]Adapted from Flexer and Savage (1992), with permission of Williams & Wilkins.

priate microphone position can cause distortion or decreased intensity of the input signal and thus negate any potential benefit of the amplifier.

5. If the headset is too large or moves around on the child's head, it can be wrapped in cloth or foam rubber to make it smaller and avoid slippage.

6. For infection control management, each child who uses the unit can have his or her own headset or foam earphone covers.

7. Reinforce to professionals and parents that the purpose of the unit is **not** to deliver a loud signal, but to deliver a **clearer** signal through the judicious positioning of the remote microphone close to the sound source.

8. The microphone also can be used to control the therapy session. For example, the microphone can be moved back and forth between the clinician and child to cue turn-taking behavior. The clinician is advised to maintain physical possession of the microphone because young children do not know where to place the microphone for an optimum signal. Children often put the microphone right on their lips (too close) or on the table (too far away).

9. Periodically, the audiologist and other team members need to consult to evaluate the hard-wired unit's effect on the previously selected outcome measures. Is progress in therapy being facilitated by the unit? Would the client benefit from additional amplification technology in different learning domains such as a personal FM system or a sound-field (classroom) amplification system?

■ APPENDIX 5F. SUGGESTED PROTOCOL FOR AUDIOLOGICAL AND HEARING AID EVALUATION[1]

Audiological Assessment

The audiological test procedures indicated are recommended for use with children in order to ensure that maximal use of residual hearing can be achieved in the Auditory-Verbal approach. A battery of audiological tests is always suggested since no single procedure has sufficient reliability to stand alone. Optimally, every aural habilitation program should have on-site audiological services, but, regardless of setting, close cooperation between audiology and therapy service providers is essential. Parents should be present for and participate in the administration of all assessment procedures to include them in this aspect of the child's care.

Procedures to Be Included in All Audiological Assessments, Regardless of Child's Age

- Case History/Parent Observation Report
- Otoscopic Inspection
- Acoustic Immittance: Tympanometry, Physical Volume Test, and Acoustic Reflexes. Cautious interpretation is recommended if the child is younger than six months.

For a Child 0–6 Months of Age, the Following Additional Tests Are Recommended

- Auditory Brainstem Response (ABR) — Alternating click and tone pip response by air conduction and by bone conduction. CAUTION: ABR should not stand alone for diagnostic purposes. Lack of response to ABR testing does not necessarily indicate an absence of usable hearing.
- Amplification and auditory learning are recommended as the first option unless special imaging (CT Scan or MRI) confirms an absence of the cochlea. Behavioral testing, amplification, and therapy are otherwise indicated before a decision of no usable hearing is made.

---

[1]Reprinted with permission of Auditory-Verbal International from *The Auricle,* 6(3), 5.

For a Child 6 Months to 2 Years of Age, the Following Tests Are Recommended

Use Behavioral Observation Audiometry (BOA) or Visual Reinforcement Audiometry (VRA) to obtain the following:

- Detection/Awareness of voice and warbled tones from 250-6000 Hz in the sound field and/or 250-8000 Hz under headphones.
- Startle response in sound field, under headphones, and by bone conduction.
- Evaluation of auditory skill development.

For a Child 2 to 5 Years of Age, the Following Tests Are Recommended

Use VRA or Conditioned Play Audiometry (CPA) to obtain the following:

- Response to pure tones from 250-12,000 Hz by air conduction, and bone conduction from 500-4000 Hz with masking (at 3½ years +).
- Speech Awareness Threshold (Speech Recognition Threshold if language development allows) using Ling Six Sounds (oo, ah, ee, sh, s, and m), body parts, speech perception tasks, or formal tests such as the WIPI.

For a Child 5 Years of Age and Older, the Following Tests Are Recommended

Use CPA or standard audiometry to obtain the following:
- Air and bone conduction, Speech Recognition and Speech/Word Identification.

Amplification Assessment

Electro-acoustic Analysis of Hearing Aids Should Be Performed

- On day of fitting.
- At 30–90 day intervals at user volume as well as full-on volume.
- Whenever a hearing aid is repaired. In addition, do a close check of internal settings.
- Whenever parental listening check or behavioral observation raises concern.

Sound-Field Aided Response

- Parents and therapists can prepare the child by teaching him or her to respond consistently to voice and the Ling Six Sounds.
- Aided measures should include: Speech Awareness or Recognition, Word Identification at 55 dB HL in quiet and, if possible, in noise; response to warbled pure tones from 250-6000 Hz wearing binaural hearing aids, or monaural measures to compare responses at each ear.

CAUTION: It is important that the aided results be evaluated in relation to the unaided audiogram. Recommended aided results for the "left corner" audiogram with optimum amplification should be in the 35–45 dB HL (ANSI) or better range at 250, 500, 1000 Hz.

Probe Microphone (Real Ear) Measures Should Include

- Uoccluded measurement of External Ear Effect as well as full occlusion with the hearing aid OFF to measure insertion loss.
- Insertion gain measured with hearing aid at customary settings to verify appropriate gain and output levels and to compare changes in settings.

CAUTION: Existing formulae may underestimate the gain required by children with severe to profound hearing impairment.

FM Systems

- When FM systems are in use, they should be evaluated at the time of the complete audiological and hearing aid assessment using the same format described for amplification.

Frequency of Assessment (Aided and Unaided)

- Every 90 days once diagnosis is confirmed and amplification fitted, until age 3.
- As early as possible, but at least by age 2, a complete unaided and aided audiogram should be obtained (preferably under headphones, but at least in the sound field.)

- New earmolds may need to be obtained at 90 day intervals or sooner until age 3–4 years in view of the typically rapid growth rate during this time.
- Assessment every 6 months from age 4–6 years is appropriate if progress is satisfactory.
- Above age 6 years, assessment at 6–12 month intervals is appropriate with earmolds at the same intervals.
- Immediate evaluation should be scheduled if parents or caretakers suspect a change in hearing or hearing aid function.

CAUTION: Modifications of this schedule are appropriate when middle ear disease is chronic or recurrent, and/or when additional disabilities are present.

Reports

Reports should be supplied promptly upon receipt of written release and sent to parents, therapists, physicians, and educators. Reports should include:

- Test procedures and reliability assessment.
- The complete audiogram with symbol key, calibration standard, and stimuli used.
- Hearing aid identification or make, model, output and tone settings, compression or special feature settings, volume setting, earmold style, and quality of fit.
- FM system identification and settings.
- Interpretive information regarding relationship of audiological findings to acoustic phonetics, especially with respect to distance hearing and message competition.
- Analysis of auditory behaviors and development of the listening function.

CAROL FLEXER ■

CATHERINE RICHARDS ■

■ CHAPTER 6

Federal Laws That Govern the Provision of Audiological Services for Infants and Children

N ow that the overwhelming necessity for hearing management leading to the development of listening skills has been presented, the audiologic services required by federal laws must be explored. Does the law support comprehensive audiologic management and hearing accessibility for *all* children with hearing impairments? The purpose of this chapter is to make parents and professionals aware of the laws that provide audiologic services to young children. Laws that govern special education are extensive and often require the expertise of a professional with a subspeciality in this area. The following is an overview of those laws to inform parents and professionals that children with hearing impairments are entitled to services as mandated by a series of federal laws.

■ OVERVIEW OF FEDERAL LAWS

Four main federal laws have evolved over the last 22 years that mandate audiologic services for infants and children: the Education for All Handicapped Children Act of 1975 (the original Public Law 94–142); an updated version of 94–142 called the Education of the Handicapped Act Amendments of 1986 (Public Law 99–457); the most recent revision called the Individuals with Disabilities Education Act (IDEA) Amendments of 1997 (Public Law 105–17); and the Rehabilitation Act of 1973 (specifically, Section 504), a civil rights act that focuses on "accessibility." All four federal laws require that children with disabilities have equal access to a free appropriate public education (FAPE).

Public Law 94–142

Public Law (PL) 94–142 (now called IDEA) also is known as the Education for All Handicapped Children Act of 1975. This law is the cornerstone of special education and provides four basic rights for children with disabilities. PL 94–142 mandates that

1. each child with a suspected disability is entitled to a thorough assessment of the nature and degree of a specific disability.
2. children with disabilities are entitled to a free and appropriate public education from the ages of 3 years through 21 years.
3. this education is to be provided by placement in the least restrictive environment (LRE), giving maximum emphasis to, whenever possible, placing the child with disabilities among children who are not disabled, a process known as mainstreaming.
4. these children are entitled to supplementary aids and services (*related services*) to ensure that their educational program as stipulated in an *Individualized Educational Program* (IEP), will be successful. The IEP is a legal, written contract, developed by the school and parents, that specifies instructional and related services needed for the child to obtain an appropriate education.

Related services are developmental, corrective, and other supportive services required to assist a child who is disabled to benefit from special education and include:

1. Transportation
2. Developmental, corrective, and other supportive services, including:
   a. audiological services
   b. speech/language therapy
   c. psychological services
   d. physical and occupational therapy
   e. recreation, including therapeutic, recreation, and social work services, and medical and counseling services (such medical services shall be for diagnostic and evaluation purposes only)

f. early identification and assessment of disabilities
g. school health services
h. parent counseling and training

PL 94–142 further protects the rights of parents and guaran-
tees *due process* in classification and program placement for the
child. Due process is a legal procedure designed to settle disagree-
ments between parents or guardians and the school district when
problems arise about any aspect of special education or related services. Due process generally is initiated by the parents of the child
with a disability when less formal solutions, like mediation, have
not worked.

One component of this extensive law pertains to audiology. As
clarified in the Code of Federal Regulations on Education, Title 34,
Section 300.13 (1986), audiology includes

(i) Identification of children with hearing loss;

(ii) Determination of the *range* (what frequencies or pitches are
involved), *nature* (sensorineural, conductive, or mixed loss), and
degree (mild, moderate, severe, profound) of hearing loss, including referral for medical or other *professional* (such as audiologists
or speech pathologists) attention for the *habilitation* (helping the
child form the basic capability to maximally use) of hearing;

(iii) Provision of habilitative activities, such as language habilitation, auditory training, speech reading (lipreading), hearing
evaluation, and speech conversation;

(iv) Creation and administration of programs for prevention of
hearing loss;

(v) Counseling and guidance of pupils, parents, and teachers
regarding hearing loss; and

(vi) Determination of the child's need for group and individual
amplification, selecting and fitting an appropriate hearing aid,
and evaluating the effectiveness of amplification. (p. 14)

The Code of Federal Regulations on Education provides two definitions that continue to apply to children who are hearing impaired. These may be found in Title 34, section 300.5 of the code
(1986). The code defines *deafness* as a "hearing impairment which is
so severe that the child is impaired in processing linguistic information through hearing, with or without amplification, which
adversely affects educational performance" (p. 12). The code further

defines *hard of hearing* as a "hearing impairment, whether permanent or *fluctuating*; such as that experienced by children with ear infections (otitis media), which adversely affects a child's educational performance but which is not included under the definition of deaf in this section" (p. 12).

Note that children with all degrees of hearing impairment, permanent or fluctuating, are entitled to audiologic rehabilitative services to support their educational performance.

IDEA Amendments of 1997—Public Law 105–17

Assuring that children with disabilities have the opportunity to be educated has evolved through laws that mandate certain educational rights. In addition, these laws have been amended twice since enactment in 1986 to address certain specific concerns that have arisen since the initial passage of Public Law 94–142.

In 1997, Public Law 105–17 (IDEA Amendments of 1997) was passed. The amendments of 1997 encompass all provisions contained in the 1986 and 1990 laws and amendments. Each reiteration of the disability law expands and strengthens previous legislation. Through all these amendments, the focus has been to

1. secure optimum educational benefit for children with disabilities,
2. provide professionals with greater flexibility in designing educational programs,
3. increase parental input in decision making for their child,
4. increase safety in school settings, and
5. consolidate discretionary programs to effectively serve children including infants and toddlers.

In addition, the 1997 amendments look closely at what educational results actually are achieved, rather than primarily at educational entitlement issues.

As stated earlier, the IDEA Amendments of 1997 do not take away any rights or services provided in earlier special education laws. However, there are two important changes that may affect how young children who are hearing impaired receive special education services.

The first important change addresses how children with disabilities are categorized. Currently, children with disabilities can be classified into 13 distinct categories, depending on the nature of their handicapping condition (e.g., autism, multihandicapped, visually impaired, hearing impaired, or developmental delay). The 1997 IDEA amendments expanded the category of "developmental delay" to allow placement of children with disabilities between the ages of 3 years through 9 years in this category rather than into a more specific disability classification. This placement may be done at the discretion of the state or local district. Because the needs of children who are hearing impaired are more specific than just general developmental issues, there is concern that these children may not receive appropriate services.

The second important change deals with the communication needs of children who are hearing impaired. Section 614(d)(3)(B)(iv) states that the

> IEP team must consider the language and communication needs of the child; opportunities for direct communication with peers and professional personnel in the child's language and communication mode, academic level, and full range of needs, including opportunities for direct instruction in the child's language and communication mode.

Provisions are also included to require that a child's need for assistive technology devices and services be addressed when developing the IEP.

Audiologists and other team members must assume an active role in the implementation of the audiology portions of Public Laws 94–142 and the IDEA amendments. In the event that an audiologist is not included on the multidisciplinary team, contact with a designated interventionist such as a speech-language pathologist or school nurse is imperative to ensure that audiologic recommendations and management are considered. Especially critical is the need for audiologists to expand their role definition from primarily diagnostic to include the provision of aural habilitative and rehabilitative services. Diagnosis without management is worthless. *Federal law supports the full spectrum of audiologic services required for hearing management for children of all ages.*

■ INDIVIDUALIZED FAMILY SERVICE PLANS (IFSPs) AND INDIVIDUALIZED EDUCATIONAL PLANS (IEPs): HOW TO MAKE HEARING SERVICES A REALITY FOR CHILDREN

The focus of this book is on infants and toddlers—from birth to 3 years of age. Under the IDEA Amendments of 1997, Part C addresses the laws that govern the provision of services to this population. The Federal government recognizes the fact that when children who have disabilities receive appropriate early intervention services and their needs are specifically addressed, then these children may not require such an intense level of special education services when they start school. To that end, states that choose to participate in at-risk programs for infants and toddlers from birth to age 3 are eligible to receive funding for their programs under Part C of the IDEA Amendments of 1997.

States that participate must designate a specific state agency that is responsible for coordinating all services for early education that are covered by Part C. Children are referred to this designated agency by hospitals, doctors, health care providers, social service providers, day care centers, or the parents themselves, for evaluation for Part C services.

According to Tucker (1998b), under Part C, infants and toddlers are entitled to the following services:

1. family training and counseling;
2. special instruction;
3. speech-language pathology and audiology services;
4. psychological services;
5. occupational and/or physical therapy;
6. service coordination services;
7. early identification, screening, and assessment services;
8. social work services;
9. assistive technology devices and accompanying services;
10. transportation and related services necessary to enable the child or the child's family to receive early intervention services;
11. health services necessary to allow the infant or toddler to benefit from other early intervention services; and
12. vision services.

Before a child can be evaluated, parents must provide written consent. Once consent has been given, the evaluation must be completed within 45 days of referral. Parents do have the option of declining the evaluation if they choose; however, the state agency has the option of initiating due process proceedings if the parents refuse. Once a child has been determined to be eligible for services, a meeting will be set up to develop an IFSP. At this point, parents have the option of refusing services under Part C without any recourse on the part of the state agency.

Ensuring that a child receives the services he or she needs and is entitled to is accomplished through the formulation of legally binding documents designed to meet federal guidelines. The two main vehicles used to establish how the child will be served are the IFSP and the Individualized Educational Plan (IEP). These two documents are of vital importance to a child's future academic success. The key word to remember in the formulation of these two plans is *individualized*. The degree to which these plans serve the specific needs of the individual child frequently establishes the educational framework that will be used to teach the child for the remainder of his or her school career. Parents have a critical responsibility to understand what their child needs and is entitled to in order to succeed academically. Unfortunately, many, if not most, parents do not understand what their child needs or how the goals and objectives stated in the IEP will be achieved. For some parents, the formulation of these plans may turn into an overwhelming experience that consists of professionals determining the content of the IEP without parental input.

Audiologists and speech-language pathologists who manage children with hearing impairment need to be knowledgeable about the types of services and accommodations they will need when he or she begins an educational program. Recommendations that are never made, obviously, can never be followed. Additionally, it is the professionals' *responsibility* to make sure that a child's parents *fully* understand information so that they can knowledgeably participate in the formation of their child's IFSP and IEP.

The Individualized Family Service Plan (IFSP)

The IFSP of the 1997 IDEA Amendments, Part C is a written, legal document that describes a plan for services for infants and toddlers and their families. An IFSP considers the child within the context of the family, is developed according to the family's priorities, and is intended to be very flexible. Dissemination of information to the family about their child's disability is a critical facet of the IFSP process. Even though an IFSP is formulated with extensive input from the child's family, Tucker (1998b) notes that it still must meet certain specific criteria. According to PL 105–17, the IFSP must include:

1. A description of the child's current level of development in the areas of physical, cognitive, communicative, psychosocial, and adaptive or self-help behaviors. These abilities usually are measured through

the use of standardized tests—tests that have reference in instruction manuals to previous research done to establish the reliability and validity of the test instrument;

2. A statement of the family's concerns, priorities, and resources as they relate to the development of their child with exceptionalities;

3. A statement of expected outcomes (goals) to be achieved for the child and family by the appropriate professionals;

4. Criteria and review/evaluation processes defined to measure progress of the child;

5. A description of the specific early intervention services that the child is to receive;

6. A description of how often the child will be seen, how long each session is, where the services will be provided (home, clinic, day care center, etc.) and method of intervention service delivery;

7. A date of initiation of services;

8. How long the child is to receive the services (e.g., 6 months, 12 months, etc.);

9. The name of the service coordinator responsible for implementing and coordinating services among agencies and professionals;

10. A description of a transition plan to appropriate preschool (Part C services to Part B) services after age 3, as necessary.

Once an IFSP has been formulated, it must be reviewed by the child's family every 6 months and evaluated on a yearly basis. Only services that the parents have consented to may be provided to the child.

Amendments to IDEA allowed IFSPs to be continued for children from ages 3 to 5 to assist them in transition to preschool programs, if the IFSP is consistent with the state policy and with the wishes of the child's parents.

If parents do not choose to continue the IFSP for a child who is between the ages of 3 to 5 and is enrolled in a preschool program that receives federal funding, an Individualized Educational Plan (IEP) must then be formulated. See Table 6–1 for required information for an IFSP, including the audiologist's role.

The Individualized Educational Plan (IEP)

The Individualized Education Plan (IEP) of the 1997 IDEA Amendments is generated when a child is identified as being unable to derive educational benefit from the standard school curriculum as

TABLE 6–1. Required Information for the IFSP and the Audiologist's Role in Contributing to That Information

Required Information	Audiologist's Role
A statement of present levels of development in the areas of physical (including vision, hearing and health), cognitive, language and speech, social-emotional, self-help.	Present results of audiological assessments, including information regarding the child's auditory development and functional use of hearing; describe the impact of the hearing impairment on communication, language, learning, and social/emotional development.
A statement of the family's resources, priorities, and concerns related to enhancing the development of the child.	Provide additional information or clarification when appropriate to support the parents and supplement the group discussion.
A statement of the major outcomes expected to be achieved for the child and the family, and the criteria, procedures, and timelines used to determine the degree to which progress toward achieving the outcomes is being made and whether or not revisions of the outcomes or services are necessary.	Assist the family in the development of the outcomes and evaluation components, especially those relevant to the child's hearing.
A statement of specific early intervention services necessary to meet the unique needs of the child and the family. This statement should reflect that there was a discussion about the options and array of community services available for the child and family.	Provide specific recommendations for intervention and treatment of the child related to the hearing impairment and the supports needed and desired by the family. Include all service and program options discussed with the family.
The projected dates for initiation of the services and the anticipated duration of the services.	Assist the family in determining these dates.
The name of the person responsible for implementing the service plan and coordinating the process among other agencies and/or persons.	Assist the family in determining who this individual will be.
The steps to be taken to support the child's transition to preschool services, if appropriate.	Help bridge the family between clinical and school-based audiology services; schedule a meeting with both audiologists and parents present to determine roles and responsibilities related to the child's audiology services needs.

Source: From *Educational Audiology Handbook,* by C. D. Johnson, P. V. Benson, and J. B. Seaton, 1997, p. 164, San Diego, CA: Singular Publishing Group. Reprinted with permission.

the result of a particular disability. Put another way, the child may demonstrate a discrepancy between ability and performance or is so severely disabled that participation in a regular education curriculum is inappropriate. Special education areas of need are targeted, and accommodations and related services are integrated into the child's school day. An IEP is supposed to be designed to enable a child with a disability to obtain an individualized, free, and appropriate public education (FAPE) in the least restrictive environment (LRE), with emphasis on that program occurring within the regular mainstream classroom.

The reason IEP issues are discussed here is because the IEP is the only ticket into the system of resource allocation that allows a child to receive any special technology, services, or strategies in school through the offices of Special Education.

All hearing services—including the availability, use, and maintenance of technology, listening strategies, and any other audiologic rehabilitative services—must be carefully detailed on the IEP or the school is under *no* obligation to provide such technology and services. Furthermore, even when the school knows and recognizes that a child needs a particular accommodation or assistive technology, unless the parent is knowledgeable enough about the needs of the child to request the service, the school is under no obligation to offer assistance. Therefore, the best of audiologic recommendations *cannot* and typically *will not* be implemented by the school unless those recommendations are incorporated into the IEP.

*As a result, the audiologist must be an active participant in the IFSP or IEP process to ensure that assistive technologies and support services are coordinated across other goals. It is not possible for a child with **any** degree of hearing impairment to obtain an appropriate education until and unless hearing is carefully and thoroughly managed* (Maddel, 1990; Ross, 1991).

All too often, for a child with a hearing impairment, the only audiologic goal specified on the IEP is that the child must have a hearing test once a year—as if assessment is an end in itself rather than a means of determining appropriate rehabilitative services. To assist an audiologist in effectively participating in an IEP conference, the following discussion will include the purpose and the components of the IEP.

Purpose of an IEP

The IEP, when developed and implemented as intended by the lawmakers, has a very positive function: the provision of *individualized* accommodations that enable a child with special needs to obtain an appropriate education. At this point, a short discussion and clarification of the word "appropriate," as it relates to and is defined by schools, is necessary. Although this word is defined as "especially suitable, or fitting," a great deal of controversy occurs between schools and parents over what is perceived to be *appropriate* and what is *ideal*. A school system does not need to provide an *ideal* education, only an appropriate one. In some school systems, preferential seating and speech therapy focusing on articulation problems once a week for 20 minutes may be viewed as *appropriate* intervention for a child who is hearing impaired; provision of assistive technology may be considered to be *ideal*. With this point of reference, bear in mind that "appropriate" is frequently a negotiable item or concept. Accordingly, no technology or special services can be provided for a child through the use of Special Education funds until those accommodations are justified and stated explicitly on the IEP.

Although an IEP serves as a blueprint for a child's educational program, this document was originally designed to serve a number of specific purposes:

1. The IEP meeting serves as a communication vehicle between parents and school personnel and enables them, as equal participants, to *jointly* decide what the child's needs are, what will be provided, and what the anticipated outcomes may be.
2. The IEP itself serves as the focal point for resolving any differences between the parents and the school, first through the meeting and second, if necessary, through the procedural projections (due process) that are available to the parents.
3. The IEP sets forth in writing a commitment of resources necessary to enable a child with disabilities to receive needed special education and related services.
4. The IEP is a management tool that is used to ensure that each child with disabilities is provided special education and related services appropriate to his or her special learning needs.
5. The IEP is a compliance/monitoring document that may be used by monitoring personnel from each government level to determine whether a child with disabilities is actually receiving the free appropriate public education agreed to by the parents and the school.

6. The IEP serves as an evaluation device for use in determining the extent of the child's progress toward meeting the projected outcomes. Methods of evaluating this progress must be included on the IEP. (*Note*: The law does not require that teachers or other school personnel be held accountable if a child with a disability does not achieve the goals and objectives set forth in his or her IEP. However, failure to achieve the goals and objectives may contribute to a parent's decision to request an Extended School Year (ESY) for their child. ESY refers to related services or an educational program that is provided for the child beyond the typical 180-day school year. Qualification criteria for ESY may vary from state to state and need to be addressed through each school district's office of special education.)

Components of an IEP

An understanding of the components of an IEP will assist the audiologist in developing appropriate and meaningful hearing related objectives. According to the amendments of 1997, the IEP shall include

1. The child's present levels of development, functioning or educational performance;
2. The annual goals for the child, including both the long- and short-term objectives;
3. A statement of how progress toward each annual goal will be measured, when and how parents will be informed of progress, and who is responsible for working on designated goals;
4. A statement of services, including related services that are needed to implement each goal;
5. An explanation of the extent to which the child will not participate with nondisabled children in the regular class and in the general education curriculum, including extracurricular and nonacademic activities;
6. A statement of any individual modifications in the administration of state and district-wide assessments;
7. The dates on which it is expected that the services listed will begin, how often the child will be served, where services will be delivered, and how long each session will last;
8. Beginning at age 14, a statement of the transition service needs of the child under the applicable compo-

nents of the child's IEP that focus on the child's course of study. (The purpose of this plan is to address how the child's educational program can be planned to help the child make a successful transition to his or her goals for life after secondary school.)

9. If appropriate, at the age of 16, a transition plan to determine what services are needed, including instruction, community experiences, the development of employment and other post school objectives, and independent living skills, if necessary.

At this point it should be stressed that the components listed above are the *minimum* elements that must be contained in the IEP. Each state sets its own requirements and parents should request a copy of those regulations from the appropriate state agency.

To summarize, in a very logical fashion the IEP specifies where the child is functioning now, where you want him or her to be functioning at the end of the school year, how you plan to achieve that long term goal, and how you can determine whether the goal was actually reached.

For example, if the child has difficulty listening in a group situation, the listening difficulty and present level of listening function need to be documented, initially, through some evaluative tool. (Tests of speech perception and auditory function are discussed in Chapter 7.) Then, a long-term plan for improving listening must be formulated, followed by the short-term steps necessary to reach the long-term goal. Finally, the means of evaluating progress toward the listening goal need to be specified. If the audiologist simply states in the recommendations section of the audiologic assessment that listening skills should be facilitated in group learning situations, there is no assurance that the IEP team can or will translate that recommendation into an appropriate behavioral objective format for inclusion in the IEP.

Another example is the use of speech-to-noise ratio enhancing equipment (assistive technology) in all instructional settings and learning domains. The *daily* use, maintenance, and *monitoring* (as mandated by PL 94–142) of all equipment must be stated specifically and precisely in the IEP or resources and personnel will not be allocated. Again, audiologists who are familiar with the dimensions of the IEP have a better chance of being successful in the meaningful integration of all amplification and assistive technologies into the child's learning environments.

An important point to bear in mind is that IFSPs and IEPs usually are formulated to provide educational intervention to children who have demonstrated a discrepancy between ability and achievement. Is the child failing badly enough to warrant intervention through placement in a special education program? Generally, children who exhibit more severe or profound forms and degrees of disabilities, such as physical or mental developmental delays, orthopedic impairment, sensory impairments of vision and hearing, or severe emotional disturbance, qualify for intervention because the impact of the disability is usually easily identified. However, there is a large population of children who are required to qualify for special education on the basis of failure in a regular classroom setting. The reason these children have to demonstrate failure before receiving help is that their disabilities are not easily recognized. Examples of these children are:

- Children who have learning disabilities secondary to minimal and/or fluctuating hearing loss,
- Children with attentional difficulties that may be related to minimal and/or fluctuating hearing loss,
- Children with auditory processing disorders that may be related to minimal and/or fluctuating hearing loss,
- Children who have *no* actual learning problems other than the 2 standard deviation discrepancy between performance and ability that may be due to minimal and/or fluctuating hearing loss.

It is not until this large population of children *fails* that intervention is remotely considered. This group of children may be eligible for help based on a fourth federal law that protects them even though qualification for special education has not been established.

Section 504 of the Rehabilitation Act of 1973

Section 504 of the Rehabilitation Act of 1973 is a civil rights act that prohibits recipients (such as agencies and organizations) of federal funds from discriminating against "qualified individuals with disabilities in the United States." Specifically, a recipient of federal funds that operates a public elementary or secondary education program shall provide a free, appropriate public education (FAPE) to each qualified person with a disability who is in the recipient's jurisdiction, regardless of the nature or severity of the person's disability.

Section 504 protects children and adults with many different kinds of physical and mental disabilities. The term disability is very broad and includes any person who (DuBow, Geer, & Strauss, 1992):

1. has a physical or mental impairment that substantially limits one or more major life activities,

2. has a record of such an impairment, or

3. is regarded as having such an impairment. (p. 51)

Major life activities include such items as the ability to take care of oneself, walking, hearing, doing manual tasks, seeing, speaking, breathing, learning, and working.

DeConde Johnson (1992) identified ways that IDEA and Section 504 of the Rehabilitation Act of 1973 can complement each other to provide comprehensive services for children with all types and degrees of auditory impairments:

1. IDEA specifies that special education and related services must be provided through an IFSP or an IEP so that a child with a disability can obtain an appropriate education, but Section 504 recognizes that an appropriate education might be provided through regular education or related aids and services without an IEP. Key words and concepts that are used in each law that can distinguish special education from regular education services are *eligibility* for special education under IDEA, compared to *protected* under Section 504. *Therefore, there are potentially many more children who may be eligible to receive services through Section 504 than who might be eligible for services under IDEA*; such children do not meet the *eligibility* criteria for special education, yet they do not have equal *access* to a free and appropriate public education (FAPE) due to an impairment.

2. School districts have an obligation to provide services (such as evaluations, regular education, reasonable accommodations, related services, and related aids) regardless of the eligibility for special education under IDEA. In other words, a school district may be obligated to use *regular education funds* to provide related services and/or aids for a child who is disabled.

3. Even though school districts provide FAPE through special education programming, such programming does not necessarily mean that the situation is in compliance with Section 504, particularly if the child receives special education services in a building or classroom segregated from the other typical students.

4. For children who experience central auditory processing disorders, attention difficulties, or *minimal* hearing impairments (such as is experienced with ear infections and otitis media), the implications of Section 504 revolve around *access to auditory information or acoustic accessibility*. Therefore, S/N ratio-enhancing technology, such as personal FM systems and sound-field FM systems, might be justified as providing acoustic accessibility without the student needing to meet the handicapping eligibility criteria for special education under IDEA. In other words, regular education (the child's school) would be responsible for furnishing the necessary amplification technology that provides accessibility to auditory information in a school environment—if it can be demonstrated that the child does *not* have access to instructional information without such technology.

5. The school must give consideration, under Section 504, to nonacademic and extracurricular services and activities as well as to academic ones. That is, the school must provide the S/N ratio-enhancing technology that would enable the child with an auditory impairment to participate in sports, school clubs, or other school-related extracurricular activities. See Appendix 6–A for an example of a Section 504 plan.

■ SUMMARY

Federal laws both mandate services and protect the rights of infants and children with disabilities. Public Law 94–142 formed the initial framework for special education and continues in effect today through the IDEA Amendments of 1997. These laws mandate the formulation of Individualized Family Service Plans (IFSPs) and Individualized Education Plans (IEPs) for children who *qualify* for special education services after the completion of a multifactored evaluation. These legally binding agreements are vehicles that ensure that the child with a disability will receive the educational services and accommodations necessary to provide him or her with access to a free, appropriate public education (FAPE).

Section 504, subpart D of the Rehabilitation Act of 1973, *protects* the rights of qualified children who are disabled by ensuring that these children have *access* to FAPE through the formulation of a 504 plan. Access is guaranteed even though the child with the disability is not being served through special education services and an existing IFSP or IEP. Provisions for children who fall under Section 504 may need to be financed by regular education funds.

Audiologists and clinicians who provide early intervention to children who have hearing problems need to be aware of and familiar with these federal laws and provide interpretation and information about them to parents. Parents must be aware of the rights their children have and know how these laws can be used to their child's advantage. The audiologist who provides adequate parental preparation about the IFSP and IEP process will help ensure that infants and children receive the proper services and technological accommodations necessary for the acquisition of academic competencies.

■ APPENDIX 6A. SAMPLE SECTION 504 INDIVIDUALIZED EDUCATIONAL PLAN[1]

Student: _____   Date: _____

Date of Birth: _____   School: _____

Date of Meeting: _____   Grade Level: _____

As a result of a special education evaluation and staffing procedure, it was determined that this student does not qualify for special education services as defined by The Individuals With Disabilities Education Act (IDEA).

Nevertheless, the school recognizes that _____ is or may experience challenges in school. Therefore, the school has agreed to modify or adapt the classroom and/or other school environments to accommodate _____ individual needs as follows by:

_____ Providing a structured learning environment by allowing the student to keep his/her desk removed from other students and providing a daily written schedule to follow the class

_____ Supplementing verbal instructions with visual instructions

_____ Using behavioral management techniques, such as _____

_____ Adjusting class schedule

_____ Modifying test delivery by _____

_____ Giving the student additional time to complete assignments

_____ Using tape recorders, computer-aided instruction, or other audiovisual equipment

_____ Selecting modified textbooks or workbooks

_____ Tailoring homework assignments

_____ Use of one-to-one peer tutors, aides, and/or note takers

_____ Involvement of a "services coordinator" to oversee implementation of these accommodations

_____ Modification of nonacademic times such as lunchroom, recess, and physical education by:

_____

_____ Use of assistive listening device

_____ Specialized seating arrangement to enhance ability to hear in the classroom

_____ Special communication strategies such as getting student's attention, facing student, speaking clearly, and speaking in close proximity to student, minimizing background noise

_____ Other: _____

_____

_____

_____

Participating Team Members:

_____   _____
Signature   Signature

_____   _____
Signature   Signature

_____   _____
Signature   Signature

---

[1]Reprinted with permission from *Educational Audiology Handbook*, by C. D. Johnson, P. V. Beeson, and J. B. Seaton, 1997, p. 452. San Diego: Singular Publishing Group.

CAROL FLEXER ■
CATHERINE RICHARDS ■

■ CHAPTER 7

Strategies for Facilitating Hearing and Listening in All Children—With or Without Hearing Loss

Children—with or without a hearing loss—are not able to "listen" like adults. The auditory neural network of a child is not as developed as that of an adult because the higher cortical areas of the brain are not fully mature until a child is about 15 years old. In addition, children do not bring years of language and world experience to a listening situation; thus, children cannot perform auditory/cognitive closure of missed information.

There are data to suggest that listening experience (having access to the language sounds in the world) also may be important for all children in terms of influencing the spatial organization and richness of their auditory cortex, especially in the early years of brain neural plasticity (Boothroyd, 1997; Musiek & Berge, 1998). If spatial organization of the auditory cortex is influenced by the properties of the acoustic environment in which an infant is raised, then enriching the auditory environment causes enrichment of the auditory brain centers (Sharpe, 1994). Therefore, sounds must be routinely and efficiently channeled into the auditory system through management of acoustic/learning environments, the judicious use of hearing aids when necessary, and S/N ratio-enhancing technology.

A child who has a hearing loss should be able to *hear* (receive sounds) better with hearing aids than without them. Unfortunately, amplification alone does not necessarily ensure that the child will be better able to *listen*, just as having "normal" hearing does not guarantee the development of listening skills, especially in children with disabilities.

195 ■

Unless a purposeful attempt is made to teach the child what to listen for, the only goal that may be achieved with amplification is to increase the volume of sounds that he or she hears. An analogy may help explain this concept. Most people who step out into their backyard or go to a park are able to hear the sounds of many different birds in the environment. However, few people would be able to identify what specific type of bird was producing a particular song or call. The ability to distinguish bird calls requires the development of a specific *listening* skill that must be learned over time and practiced frequently. Undoubtedly, it may be possible for some people to learn the differences between a few bird calls through general experience; however, this is not "proficiency." Generally, the only people who are truly proficient at differentiating and knowing the calls of many birds, are ornithologists and some highly dedicated amateur birdwatchers. The goal in teaching listening skills to children who have hearing problems is to make them as proficient listeners as possible.

A child must be provided with opportunities to learn the meaning of incoming sounds. The focus is not on pointless, isolated auditory training sessions that occur twice weekly for 20 minutes, but rather on integrating listening skills and spoken communication into daily life; i.e., auditory *living*, not mere auditory training. Listening skills are not separate from learning, but are the means of learning.

This chapter discusses issues and strategies related to the facilitation of auditory skills for all infants and children, whether or not they have a hearing loss. Accordingly, the following topics are addressed: levels of auditory skill development, tests of auditory/speech perception, and guidelines for maximizing hearing and facilitating listening in infants and young children.

■ LEVELS OF AUDITORY SKILL DEVELOPMENT

Erber (1982) specified a hierarchy of auditory skill development that is very helpful in understanding the evolution of auditory processing capabilities. This hierarchy has been elaborated by Estabrooks (1994; 1998); Ling (1989); and Pollack, Goldberg, and Caleffe-Schenck (1997). The initial level is *detection*, which is the ability to determine the presence or absence of sound. Detection occurs when sounds are received through an individual's sensory receptors such as the hair cells in the inner ear, and the acoustic stimuli subsequently are recognized as sensation by the person receiving the sound input. Therefore, the child learns to pay attention to sound—to respond when sound is present and not to respond when there is no sound. A child's response to the pure tones used in audiometric testing is an example of a detection task.

The next level of auditory skill development is *discrimination*. Discrimination is the ability to distinguish differences between sounds, that is, differences in sound qualities, intensities, duration, and/or pitches.

The next level is *identification*, the ability to recognize a speech stimulus and to label or name what has been heard by repeating, pointing to, or writing the word or sentence that has been perceived. The identification level involves both suprasegmental and segmental aspects of speech. *Suprasegmentals* include the prosodic elements of speech such as duration (long versus short sounds), rate (fast and slow sounds), pitch (high and low pitches), intensity (soft and loud sounds), and stress (changes in stress patterns). *Segmentals* are individual speech sounds or phonemes such as b, m, s, etc.

The last, and highest, level of auditory skill development is *comprehension*—the ultimate goal of auditory processing. Comprehension is the ability of an individual to understand the meaning of acoustic messages by references to his or her knowledge of language. Comprehension can be demonstrated by skills such as following oral directions, answering questions about a story, paraphrasing a story, giving the opposite of a word, and communicating appropriately. Comprehension necessitates the skills of auditory memory and sequencing.

Comprehension of acoustic messages cannot occur unless and until the child has attained skills in the previous three auditory levels. For example, a teacher in an early intervention program called an audiologist because a 3-year-old child with Down syndrome who was enrolled in the program appeared to be having difficulty comprehending spoken communication. The child responded inconsistently to her name and to simple commands. The teacher was concerned that the child might have auditory processing problems. When the teacher was questioned about the child's hearing sensitivity, it was discovered that the child had a long history of ear infections and was under a physician's care. There was no information about which speech sounds the child could detect. Moreover, there was no ongoing information about how the child's detection capabilities varied over time and with the presence of ear infections. Team members were focusing on the child's comprehension skills to the exclusion of prerequisite conditions. *Thus, even though auditory comprehension is the ultimate goal, without the initial detection of individual speech sounds, none of the higher levels of auditory processing can occur.*

An important fact to bear in mind when determining the hearing sensitivity of infants and young children is that a precise measure of hearing sometimes can be obtained only with repeated hearing tests. Management of the child with a hearing impairment must be based on current audiologic information that is constantly updated as additional information is documented. It is important for the audiologist to begin a flexible intervention plan immediately, rather than wait until he or she feels that test results are stable. Auditory intervention can be started as *soon* as a hearing problem is identified, and then modified as more information becomes known. Assessment without management equals time wasted.

■ TESTS OF AUDITORY PERCEPTION

Several tests are available to assist in the evaluation of a young child's auditory skill at various levels of auditory development. Examples of such tests are: Meaningful Auditory Integration Scale for Infants and Toddlers (IT-MAIS), Sound Effects Recognition Test (SERT), Early Speech Perception Test (ESP), Auditory Numbers Test (ANT), The Minimal Auditory Capabilities Battery (MAC BATTERY), Glendonald Auditory Screening Procedure (GASP), Test of Auditory Comprehension (TAC), Children's Auditory Test (CAT), The Auditory Perception of Alphabet Letters (APAL), Word Intelligibility by Picture Identification (WIPI), and the Northwestern University Children's Perception of Speech (NU-CHIPS). See Table 7–1 for a summary of each test and refer to Appendix 7-A for more detailed information.

TABLE 7–1. Tests of Auditory Skill Development

Test Name	Skill Evaluated
Auditory Numbers Test (ANT)	Evaluates the child's ability to perceive spectral aspects or only gross temporal acoustic patterns.
The Auditory Perception of Alphabet Letters (APAL)	The child listens to the names of letters from an audiotape and picks the correct one from a closed-set format. The test score is weighted according to how close acoustically the response is to the correct answer.

(continued)

TABLE 7–1. *(continued)*

Test Name	Skill Evaluated
Children's Auditory Test (CAT)	Evaluates the child's speech perception ability to determine whether he or she can make use of spectral cues to demonstrate exact word identification abilities and/or use suprasegmental cues in the identification of stress patterns only.
Early Speech Perception Test (ESP)	Designed for children with limited vocabulary and language skills. Words presented are known by the majority of 6-year-old children who are hearing impaired and may be identified by children who are unable to read.
Glendonald Auditory Screening Procedure (GASP)	Evaluates the listening skills using three subtests. The child's performance is described both in terms of what the child perceives and the adaptive strategies that can be used to help the child succeed.
Meaningful Auditory Integration Scale for Infants and Toddlers (IT-MAIS)	A parent interview format using a 4-point rating scale of auditory and device behaviors that provides valuable information regarding cochlear implant candidacy and hearing aid and/or cochlear implant benefit in very young children.
The Minimal Auditory Capabilities Battery (MAC BATTERY)	Used for the profound postlingually deaf. Consists of 13 subtests and a speech reading test.
Northwestern University Children's Perception of Speech (NU-CHIPS)	A discrimination test for children as young as 3 years of age. The child identifies pictures from a closed set by pointing to the correct item as he or she hears it.
Sound Effects Recognition Test (SERT)	Tests sound effects recognition using environmental stimuli. The child points to the picture that goes with each sound.
Test of Auditory Comprehension (TAC)	Assesses auditory function and provides a profile of the child's auditory skills in the areas of discrimination, memory sequencing, and figure-ground.
Word Intelligibility by Picture Identification (WIPI)	Tests a child's word recognition ability using six pictures per plate. The child points to a word as the tester uses a carrier phrase "show me" preceding each word.

Note: Complete references for tests may be found in Appendix 7-A.

There are additional tests that can assist in the evaluation of an infant's overall development and in a young child's development of receptive and oral expressive language behaviors: Developmental Activities Screening Inventory (DASI II), the SKI*HI Language Development Scale (LDS), Preschool Language Scale-3 (PLS-3), BOEHM Test of Basic Concepts—Preschool Version, Bracken Basic Concept Scale—Revised (BBCS-R), Test of Word Knowledge (TOWK), Peabody Picture Vocabulary Test—Revised (PPVT-R), Structured Photographic Expressive Language Test—Preschool (SPELT-P), Test of Auditory Comprehension of Language—Revised (TACL-R), and the Ling Phonetic Level Evaluation (PLE). Refer to Table 7–2 for an overview and to Appendix 7-A for more detailed information.

Note that the child's ability to *hear* the test material must be known and then maximized prior to administration of any test. An audiologic evaluation should be performed *before* any auditory or language tests are given. Interpretation of a child's higher levels of auditory and linguistic skills is impossible without knowing the child's peripheral hearing sensitivity. For more information about the use of assessment tools for listening skills and auditory-receptive abilities, please refer to Edwards (1991); Estabrooks (1994; 1998); and Ross, Brackett, and Maxon (1991).

TABLE 7–2. Tests of Overall Development and Receptive/Expressive Language Behaviors

Test Name	Skills Evaluated
Boehm Test of Basic Concepts—Preschool Version	Measures child's knowledge of 26 basic relational concepts, such as up, all, under, that are necessary for achievement in school. The examiner shows the child pictures, and he or she points to that portion that answers the examiner's questions.
Bracken Basic Concept Scale—Revised (BBCS-R)	This norm- and criterion-referenced scale for children, ages 2½ to 8, assesses a child's receptive knowledge of over 300 basic concepts in 11 distinct conceptual categories.
Developmental Activities Screening Inventory (DASI-II)	Informal nonverbal developmental screening for children functioning between 0 to 60 months of age. Tests a variety of skills that represent behaviors frequently included in tests of early development.

(continued)

TABLE 7–2. (continued)

Test Name	Skills Evaluated
Peabody Picture Vocabulary Test—Revised (PPVT–R)	Measures a child's receptive (hearing) vocabulary. Child points to correct picture from a plate of four pictures following examiner's request to "Show me _____ "
Phonetic Level Evaluation (PLE)	An evaluation procedure used in conjunction with Ling's text, *Speech and the Hearing Impaired Child: Theory and Practice*, on speech training for children who are hearing impaired. Evaluates nonsegmental and segmental aspects of speech. Targets are elicited by imitation of the examiner. Provides teacher or clinician with clearly defined teaching goals.
Preschool Language Scale—3 (PLS–3)	This is a two part auditory comprehension and expressive communication test. It is used as a diagnostic and screening instrument to systematically appraise the early stages of language development. Skills are positioned at age levels that represent the point at which most children have achieved competency.
The SKI*HI Language Development Scale (LDS)	Assesses expressive and receptive language skills of the child who is hearing impaired. Does not emphasize auditory items or penalize children using total communication. Administered by the parent to evaluate the child's communication skills by looking for the items in the list that the parent advisor selects.
Structured Photographic Expressive Language Test—Preschool (SPELT–P)	A screening instrument to identify children who are experiencing difficulty in their expression of early developing morphological and syntactic features.
Test of Auditory Comprehension of Language—Revised (TACL–R)	Provides an inventory of grammatical forms for observing a child's auditory comprehension behavior. No oral response is required. The student points to the picture he or she believes matches the stimulus read aloud by the examiner.
Test of Word Knowledge (TOWK)	Evaluates deficits in semantic knowledge of children, ages 5 through 17. Designed for use as part of a total diagnostic language battery, TOWK evaluates the child's ability to understand and use words.

Note: Complete references for tests may be found in Appendix 7–A.

■ GUIDELINES FOR MAXIMIZING HEARING AND FACILITATING LISTENING

Many auditory strategies can be employed by habilitation specialists; these strategies are incorporated into communicative interactions to teach the child to use his or her listening abilities in natural and meaningful situations. A philosophy that epitomizes the development of auditory potential in children with any degree of hearing impairment is *Auditory-Verbal*. The goal of auditory-verbal practice is for children with hearing impairment to grow up in regular learning and living environments that enable them to become independent, participating, and contributing citizens in mainstream society. Appendix 7-B of this chapter describes auditory-verbal practice. Many of the guidelines discussed here were derived from auditory-verbal principles.

Additional examples and specific strategies for maximizing auditory potential can be found in the following sources: Beebe (1953); Berg (1987); Clark (1989); Cole and Gregory (1986); Erber (1982); Ernst (1997); Estabrooks (1994; 1998); Estabrooks and Edwards (1986); Estabrooks and Schwartz (1995); Goldberg (1987, 1993); Ling (1989); Manning, Flexer, and Shackelford (1991); Nevitt and Brelsford (1987); Parents and Families of Natural Communication, Inc. (1998); Pollack (1985); Pollack, Goldberg, & Caleffe-Schenck (1997); Ross, Brackett, and Maxon (1982, 1991); Sindrey (1997); and Vaughn (1981).

Following are guidelines for facilitating listening in infants and children at risk for hearing loss. These guidelines are directed to parents, clinicians, and teachers—to anyone who uses spoken communication as a means of imparting information to children.

The guidelines are divided into three areas that address specific issues of concern and present strategies to facilitate the acquisition of listening skills in young children.

These areas are:

1.   Professional and medical prerequisites for initiation of intervention and therapy,
2.   Management of noise in the learning environment, and
3.   Structure of the learning environment including strategies for facilitating listening skills.

These guidelines are presented with the goal of creating an "auditory world" for infants and toddlers to allow for meaningful and ongoing stimulation of critical auditory brain centers.

Professional and Medical Prerequisites for the Initiation of Intervention and Therapy

To ensure that the child has maximum use of hearing and access to sounds, the following events must occur:

Audiologic Recommendations

A *pediatric* audiologist should be an active, contributing member of every early intervention team. The emphasis on pediatric is important because intervention for young children depends on a thorough knowledge of the child's physical, cognitive, and language development. Under IDEA, (see Chapter 6), parents are permitted to have professionals of their choosing participate in the formulation of their child's intervention plan. A pediatric audiologist's participation ensures that the child will have an advocate who is familiar with the accommodations the child requires to learn successfully. Unfortunately, most early intervention teams do not even have an audiologist present to explain the problems of a child who has hearing difficulties or even to raise the question of whether hearing should be considered in the evaluation of a child.

An example of how hearing was not considered in one child's intervention plan occurred in a developmental preschool where most of the qualifying children had language goals included on their IEPs or IFSPs. A young child who was enrolled in the class had a very obvious visual impairment as evidenced by the very thick glasses he wore. When the preschool teacher was questioned about the cause of the visual impairment, the teacher explained that the child's mother had rubella during the first trimester of her pregnancy. The second question asked was, "Does he have any hearing problems?" The teacher stated that the child had a mild hearing loss but it was *not significant*. Obviously, this intervention team which included a psychologist, a speech/language pathologist, a teacher, and a parent had never considered that hearing was an issue in this child's development. Nothing was being done to provide management of the educational problems that he probably was experiencing as a result of his mild hearing loss. Needless to say, an audiologist was not a member of this team; this child was being forced to function with unnecessary barriers. Recommendations that could have been made by an educational audiologist following a thorough audiological assessment include:

1. Sound-field amplification for the developmental preschool classroom or provision of a personal FM system to provide acoustic accessibility to the teacher's instruction. Hearing aids might also be necessary.

2. Intensive auditory and listening skill activities provided by the speech/language pathologist in addition to already existing language goals.
3. Inservicing of the classroom teacher to provide suggestions for adaptations that might be necessary to ensure that the child has an appropriate acoustic environment for learning.

Medical Recommendations

If a medical referral has been made, do everything possible to facilitate medical treatment (usually for an ear infection or removal of ear wax). Remember, physicians are trained to deal with pathology, whereas audiologists are educated to deal with the hearing impairment caused by the pathology. Neither professional can substitute for the other. Avoid the tendency to believe that if a child is under medical management, somehow the hearing loss caused by the pathology does not count. Parents should not hesitate to suggest that they are receptive to more aggressive medical measures than repeated courses of antibiotics and a "wait and see" attitude.

Audiologists who are employed by physicians need to be especially vigilant about their responsibility toward their young patients. In the interest of time and due to limited technical setups (not all offices have access to sound-field testing), thorough examination of children is sometimes not possible. Nevertheless, the audiologist *is* responsible for audiologic management recommendations, regardless of the audiologist's work setting.

For example, a young child was seen in a physician's office at the insistence of her mother because the child was experiencing significant problems, bordering on failure, in school, and there were concerns about the numerous articulation errors that were present in the child's speech. This child had a long history of middle ear infections which had prompted referral by the pediatrician to an otolaryngologist. Testing in the physician's office indicated that the child had a moderate-to-severe, bilateral, high-frequency hearing loss. The SRT was obtained at 15 dB HL. No impedance test was performed. The physician advised the parent that the hearing loss was "not significant" because it was in the high frequencies; and that nothing could be done about it. Because tympanometry was not performed, the absence of middle ear involvement was ruled out on the basis of otoscopic inspection. The audiologist briefly counseled the parent that there were some sounds the child would have difficulty hearing and that "maybe" she would benefit from an assistive listening device. However, educational problems and management strategies were never discussed with the parent, nor were any recommendations made to the school. No recommendations were made to the parent even to have the child retested. The parent left the office totally overwhelmed because she had virtually no information about what to do next.

Two days later, tympanometry was performed as part of a school hearing screening. Results indicated extreme negative pressure bilaterally and reduced thresholds as a result of an ear infection. The speech/language pathologist called the audiologist who then requested that the parent call the office for an appointment. The child was seen the next week and subsequently put on antibiotic therapy. Unfortunately, the "insignificant" high-frequency hearing loss became an "insignificant" mild-to-moderate conductive hearing loss in the low frequencies and continued to be moderate-to-severe in the high frequencies; still no educational management strategies were suggested by the audiologist. This was a cycle that repeated itself frequently for this particular child. Is it any wonder that the child was experiencing extreme behavioral and academic difficulty in school?

Any hearing impairment must be audiologically managed in conjunction with medical management of the causal pathology. *There is no such thing as an insignificant hearing impairment!*

Use of Amplification

Whenever amplification is used, intervention team members need to understand what the settings on the hearing aids or FM systems should be and the proper use of each device. At least one individual on the team should be thoroughly inserviced to perform trouble-shooting strategies. Frequently school personnel voice their opinion that equipment management should be the responsibility of the child's parents not the school. What most schools do not realize is that the IDEA Amendments of 1997 mandate that each public agency should ensure that hearing aids worn in school by children who are deaf or hard of hearing are functioning properly. Even if parents conscientiously check their child's hearing aid each morning before he or she goes to school, the school still has the responsibility of performing daily listening checks. Problems such as dead batteries, both in the child's hearing aid and in personal FM systems, can occur suddenly. Dead batteries cause the child to sit the remainder of the day in school with no amplification because no one at school has checked to see whether the hearing aids and FM units are functioning properly.

In addition, the speech sounds that the child can detect with and without amplification should be clearly understood by the intervention team. Understanding what sounds the child can and cannot hear may help explain why the child needs and must use amplification at all times.

Understanding the Role of Audition in Language Development

Parents and professionals need to be sensitized to the critical role of audition in the development of spoken communication. As mentioned earlier in Chapter 1, many people, including teachers, principals, psychologists, and even some physicians, assume that a person is either deaf or that he or she can hear normally. This belief presents an enormous problem because, unless professionals and the child's family understand the extent to which the child is disabled, intervention strategies risk being sabotaged through inconsistent management and poor follow-through of amplification recommendations.

The education of professionals can be accomplished by well-planned inservices provided throughout the school year (Ross, 1991). Parents can be counseled on an as-needed basis if the child is enrolled in an intervention program. The counseling should be provided by a clinician who is familiar with strategies and techniques used in the habilitation of children who have hearing problems.

Commercially prepared materials are an invaluable aid in helping to illustrate the effects of a hearing impairment. Three audiotapes, in particular, are useful in helping parents and professionals understand the types of difficulty children with hearing impairment experience when they hear speech. These tapes are:

1. "Sound Hearing or . . . Hearing What You Miss" by S. Harold Collins (1989), Garlic Press
2. "Getting Through, A Guide to Understanding" Self Help for Hard of Hearing People, Inc (1992).
3. "Say What . . . ? An Introduction to Hearing Loss" American Academy of Audiology (1992).

For example, a school psychologist, with many years of experience, requested a hearing screening for a student as part of a multifactored learning disability evaluation. The student failed the screening. Further testing indicated the presence of a moderate, high-frequency hearing loss bilaterally. The student used no amplification or assistive listening systems. When he was questioned about whether he had ever had hearing problems, his reply was, "Yes, I used to wear hearing aids when I was in about third grade." He did not know why he quit wearing them but suggested that maybe his mother would know. Examination of his cumulative school file did not show *any* record of hearing loss. Surprisingly, hearing loss was never considered to be a factor in this child's educational program even though he had been receiving special education services since the second grade. An explanation of what this student was able to hear and/or not hear was given to the school psychologist. An audio-tape of filtered speech was used to further illustrate the type of speech he heard on a daily basis. The psychologist was amazed at the level of difficulty this student was experiencing. The multifactored evaluation indicated that the child no longer qualified for special education services, but as a result of this demonstration and the psychologist's increased understanding of the problem he was having, the intervention team granted an override in procedure and maintained the level of service that the child had been receiving. The child's mother was then counseled to have her son's hearing evaluated, because this had not been done for five years, to determine audiological recommendations for educational management. Educational audiological recommendations that should have been made for management of this older child include:

1. Obtaining a complete, updated audiologic evaluation to determine hearing sensitivity, including speech-in-noise testing to determine what type of difficulty he may have in a classroom setting. A hearing aid evaluation should also be performed.
2. Use of a personal FM system to provide accessibility to classroom instruction.
3. Speech-language evaluation to determine higher level language abilities such as multiple word meanings, figurative language, and inference and conclusion.
4. Inservicing of teachers and tutors to provide adaptations to ensure that:
   a. notes taken on all orally presented material are complete;
   b. the child is not graded on material presented through films and tapes unless it is ascertained that his notes are complete or that he has access to captioning for the audiovisual equipment; and
   c. new vocabulary and concepts are pretutored in the resource room prior to their introduction in the classroom.

A second example involves a young child who was diagnosed with a moderate-to-severe high-frequency hearing loss. At the time of the diagnosis, the parents had no comprehension of how this problem would affect their child's long-range development. Moreover, they did not know that the reason her speech was characterized by numerous distortions and misarticulations was a direct result of her inability to hear the high-frequency speech sounds. Subsequent counseling provided by the school speech/language pathologist and the playing of the filtered speech audiotape clearly illustrated to the parents the difficulty their child was experiencing in everyday life. Because the parents now understood how their child heard, they were receptive to recommendations for hearing aids and therapy and to the purchase of a personal FM system. *Awareness precedes action.*

Management of Noise in the Learning Environment

Professionals generally refer to school classrooms and therapy rooms as learning environments because formal instruction and/or intervention is carried out there. However, a child's learning environment is, realistically, anyplace he or she gains new knowledge or information. Infants and very young children spend almost all their time at home. Therefore, the home must be considered their primary learning environment. Because children do not have the awareness to indicate that they are unable to hear or understand speech due to interfering noise, parents must be conscious of how to manage noise.

Management of noise does not imply that the child with a hearing impairment must be isolated in a sound-treated room any time someone wants to communicate with him or her. However, it does mean that, to optimize the child's learning through the auditory channel, certain conditions must exist, particularly when direct instruction is being provided.

Some suggestions for noise management in an infant or young child's home include making the environment as quiet as possible. Eliminate competing sounds by:

- Turning off radios and television sets.
- Closing a window next to a noisy area such as busy streets or when neighbors are mowing lawns.
- Turning off noisy appliances such as dryers, mixers, blenders and video games rather than trying to speak to the child over them.
- Working with the child at a time of day when noise from the other members of the family is at a minimum, (e.g., try not to plan a lesson when older siblings are

due to arrive home from school or when their play-
mates are over and require parental supervision).
- Encouraging grandparents and other relatives who
  may be babysitters or caretakers for the child to follow
  the same type of noise management suggestions.
- Speaking at a normal conversational level of loudness
  at close range rather than talking loudly from across
  the room. Yelling from a distance may promote audibility but it does not ensure or facilitate the reception of
  intelligible speech.

As the young child approaches the age when parents begin to
consider preschool, careful observation of the type of learning environment the child will be placed in is important. Parents should be
encouraged by the audiologist or clinician to visit different schools to
see classrooms firsthand and determine whether they are appropriate
before making a final placement decision. School classrooms are noto-
riously poor acoustic environments, primarily because the majority of
them were constructed to be durable and functional without consideration of the listening environment. (Berg, Blair, & Benson, 1996).

Parents should observe the classroom during the school day to
gain a sense of what the room sounds like when it is full of children.
Noise levels are an important factor in determining how the child with
hearing problems will be able to learn. Even with technology such as
personal FM systems, some environments are just not conducive to
learning because of poor speech-to-noise ratios (see Chapter 5 for
acoustic guidelines).

Factors that influence the level of noise in a school classroom
are listed below. Parents should be taught to observe what types
of measures have been taken, if any, to manage noise in the learning environment.

1.   What is the construction of the floor and ceiling in the
classroom? The floor and ceiling areas comprise 60% of the total
area of a school classroom and have an enormous impact on the
noise levels in the classroom (Ross, 1991). Observe whether:

- the classroom has carpeting, wood or tiled floors,
- the ceiling has acoustical tile or is plain plaster,
- the ceiling is less or more than 12 feet high.

*Rooms with hard floors and high ceilings will be much more
reverberant and noisy than a carpeted room with acoustical tile
and lower ceilings.*

2. Where is the classroom located in the school? Rooms across
from or adjacent to cafeterias and gymnasiums or next to busy

streets, loading docks, and playgrounds may have constantly high levels of external noise that are virtually impossible to control.

3. Does the philosophy of the school determine the classroom setup? Some schools advocate an open classroom environment with no walls between different teaching groups. Noise in open classrooms travels freely from area to area, making it difficult for children with normal hearing to hear. Children who have hearing problems need optimal speech-to-noise ratios to learn and would have an even more difficult time.

4. Does the classroom have sound-field amplification? Children who are at risk for academic failure because of minimal and/or fluctuating hearing loss, mild-to-moderate sensorineural hearing losses who are aided, unilateral hearing loss, and children with auditory processing or attentional difficulties but normal peripheral hearing benefit from sound-field amplification (see Chapter 5).

5. What is the instructional style of the teacher? Is she or he very soft-spoken or a very loud speaker? Does he or she maintain discipline by yelling at the students? How does the class function under this teacher's charge—noisy, quiet, relaxed, calm, self-guided, and so on?

6. A final consideration is the makeup of the students in the class. Most early intervention programs require that the child qualify for placement in a developmental preschool on the basis of a deficit in one or more areas of development (see Chapter 6). Placement for a child may then be recommended in a class comprised solely of children who require extensive intervention and support. Alternatively, placement may be recommended in an "integrated" setting that has children with no developmental problems attending the same class as children with various disabilities. It is altogether possible that a small special education class of 7 to 8 students could be noisier than a mainstreamed class of 15 students. Parents, under the guidance of the audiologist and/or clinician must make a personal decision whether their child will receive the support he or she needs in a special education setting or whether a mainstreamed preschool would be more beneficial and fit the family's philosophy more closely. *Only direct observation of the classroom by the parent can answer this question.*

Structure of the Learning Environment and Strategies for Facilitating Listening Skills

Facilitation of listening skills can begin after (a) the child has been provided with appropriate amplification, (b) all ear-related medical considerations have been determined and managed, and (c) the child's primary learning environment has been controlled for noise. The primary responsibility for guiding the parents, families, and teachers in listening facilitation belongs to the educational audiologist or clinician who is spearheading the aural habilitation of the child.

Information, illustrated by examples, must be conveyed to the parent about what sounds their child is and is not able to hear with his or her hearing aids. For example, "Timmy should be able to hear a toy drum, a rattle, and a squeaky toy if the room is quiet and you stand behind him no farther away than 3 or 4 feet." This information will enable the parents to have realistic and concrete knowledge on which to structure initial listening experiences for the child. Finally, because some, if not most, parents may feel overwhelmed at the enormity of the task they are undertaking, care must be exercised so that their expectations are tempered and based on small progressive steps rather than unrealistic leaps and bounds. Giving parents specific time lines should be discouraged because what one child responds to in 3 weeks may take another 8 to 10 weeks and a third child 4 months.

Parents must recognize that the initial and primary focus of listening strategies is on facilitating auditory input, not on demanding oral expressive output.

Habilitationists need to be cognizant of the different variables that affect the listening process so that they and the parents can adapt their intervention strategies effectively. These variables will be discussed relative to how the clinician and parent should affect their use. These are divided into two groups of factors by Estabrooks (1994, 1998) and by Ling (1989): linguistic factors and other factors.

Linguistic Factors

Linguistic factors include *speech sound production features,* and *suprasegmentals clues* such as stress, rate, and loudness.

Speech Sound Production Features

Even though intervention focuses on input and not on oral expressive output, once the child has had time to hear and experience the sounds of his or her world, it is inevitable that the child will begin to vocalize. If the baby or child voluntarily makes sounds, imitate those sounds. Reinforce the child's verbal behaviors by pointing to your ear and saying, "I heard you," and then respond appropriately to the intent of the utterance. For example, the child looks to the parent with raised arms and vocalizes, "uh." The parent points to her ear and says, "I heard you. 'uh,' I want up!" Then the parent picks up the child. *By emphasizing that the child's request was heard, the parent reinforces the auditory signal, not the visual gesture of raised arms.*

The child's ability to respond to the *Ling Six Sound Test (m, ah, oo, ee, sh, s)* is an important measure of how well he or she is able to hear speech sounds across the range of frequencies and how well the auditory system (hearing plus hearing aid) is working (Ling, 1989, 1997). When the child is developing and learning language utilizing an auditory approach, he or she must learn to respond to these six sounds at different distances. Conditioning the child to respond to most of these sounds can be done by incorporating them into everyday situations so that the sounds become familiar to the child. For example, a parent can say, "*mmmmmmm*, this ice cream tastes good," "*ooooo*, you scraped your knee," "*aaaaah*, that puppy is so cute," "*eeeeee*, that water's cold," or "*ssssh*, the baby is sleeping, time to be quiet." Continued conditioning then can be achieved by using rings or blocks and having the child learn to put them into a box or bucket as he or she hears the sound.

Parents also should be encouraged to sing, chant nursery rhymes, and play peek-a-boo and pattycake games. Songs and rhymes provide meaningful opportunities to enhance the suprasegmental structure of spoken language for children with all degrees of hearing impairment. The sense of rhyme and knowledge of nursery rhymes that young children develop also has been determined to be an important factor in their initial success in learning to read because rhyming is associated with phonological awareness (Bryant, Bradley, MacLean, & Crossland, 1989; Gilbertson & Bramlett, 1998).

Sentence Structure (Syntax)

Clinicians and parents should always speak in complete sentences using intonation to mark the boundaries between units of meaning. For the child to learn the linguistic rules that govern word order and word agreement, he or she must be exposed to properly constructed sentences. Children cannot model what they have not heard. Properly constructed sentences do not have to be complex; however they should be age-appropriate relative to the child's degree of language development.

Semantics (Word and Sentence Meaning, Content)

Speak to the child with a *varied* vocabulary. Use different words to convey concepts. For example, a pancake can be large, big, huge, gigantic, or even enormous; houses can be dingy, run down, tidy, beautiful, colorful, or just plain blue. The comprehension and use of the different shades of meaning can be developed only by exposure to many different words. Cultivate the use of adjectives, adverbs, synonyms, antonyms, and analogies whenever appropriate.

Pragmatics

Pragmatics refers to the social rules of how the child uses language. Parents probably can understand this most easily in the context of "manners." For example, does the child have turn-taking skills or does he or she interrupt inappropriately regardless of who is speaking. Many of the pragmatic social rules are learned through casual observation of different behaviors that occur in various settings. *Because of the inability of children who are hearing impaired to "overhear" the subtle exchanges that constantly occur between people, these children purposefully must be taught what is appropriate and what is not.* Initially, these skills can be developed by engaging the infant or child in frequent sound play games that encourage turn-taking during meaningful social interactions. As the child grows older, the game can progress from specific sounds to word productions (see Figure 7–1).

Children also can be taught to take turns by playing a simple game where a ball is passed back and forth between the listener and the speaker. When the child has the ball, he or she is the speaker and the person without the ball is the listener. Allow the infant or child sufficient time to respond to his or her conversational turn or to questions. If necessary, try counting to 8 or 10 before expecting an answer from the child or speaking again.

Managing Other Factors That Affect the Listening Process

USE CONTEXT CLUES. Context clues give the listener a sense of predictability about the types of words that may be used in the course of a conversation. Knowledge of the topic also provides context clues that serve to limit the word choices that are relevant to a particular situation. Even if the listener is unfamiliar with an individual word, he or she may gain a sense of the word's meaning when it is used in a sentence because of the surrounding words.

Young children's experiences with different situations provide settings or context-relevant vocabulary which help them generalize to other similar situations. For example, a youngster in a play situation making mud pies can learn about mixing, adding, stir-

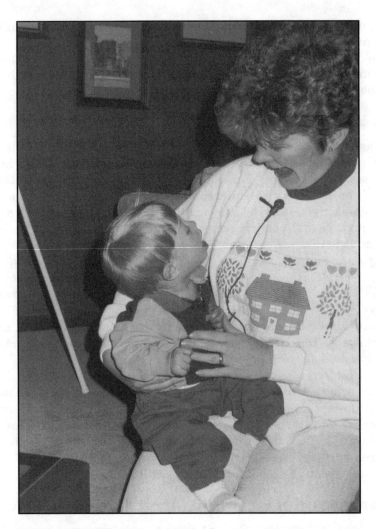

Figure 7–1. Using an FM sound-field system (with a single loudspeaker), this toddler is surrounded by sound as he and his mother engage in vocal play and singing.

ring, patting, rolling, spreading, or sprinkling. Later on, while helping or watching in the kitchen as a parent makes a real pie or cake, many of the same words may apply and would be familiar because they had been used in another context.

Clinicians and parents therefore should provide the child with meaningful contexts for repetitious learning experiences. Remem-

ber, months of interactive listening input with many different peo-
ple in a variety of settings are necessary before listening skills can
be generalized across learning domains.

Focus on integrating listening skills into daily life by talking
to the child about routine situations that relate the shared experiences of the parent and child. These experiences set situational
contexts for the child. Keep in mind that young children function
best on concrete levels. Therefore, follow the child's attention; communicate initially about the child's immediate interest. Stick to
the concrete here and now rather than trying to be abstract and
overly informative. Young attention spans are very short, so maximize the moment.

USE CLEAR SPEECH AND ACOUSTIC HIGHLIGHTING. Encourage parents,
teachers, and family members to use *clear speech* when communicating (Sindrey, 1997; Tye-Murray, 1998). Clear speech is speech
that uses a moderately loud conversational level, is characterized by
precise but not exaggerated articulation, pauses at appropriate linguistic boundaries, and uses a somewhat slow speaking rate. It is
very important for meaning, melody, and clarity to speak in sentences and not in single words.

A variation of clear speech is called *acoustic highlighting* (Estabrooks, 1994, 1998). Acoustic highlighting is speaking in such a way
that the child's chances of understanding what is said are increased.
Acoustic highlighting includes prompting the child to listen prior to
initiating a conversation; use of exaggerated and animated intonation—almost sing-song in the beginning; use of stress in a natural way
to highlight the key word to be processed; use of a reduced rate, but
not too slow or choppy; use of "auditory space"—pause briefly before
the key word; and be sure to give the child time to respond.

ENHANCE THE PROMINENCE OF THE SIGNAL BY IMPROVING THE S/N RATIO.
The speech-to-noise ratio (S/N ratio) needs to be enhanced in all
spoken communicative interactions to maximize intelligibility,
increase the redundancy of the speech signal, and focus the infant
or toddler's attention on auditory input. Be mindful of appropriate
positioning. The talker should be as close as possible to the child;
this allows speech to be directed into the baby's ear (approximately
6 inches from the ear) or into the microphone of an assistive listening device (personal FM unit, sound-field amplification, or mild
gain hard-wired unit). (See Figure 7–2 for demonstration of this
technique.)

Additionally, a parent, teacher, or clinician can use the remote
microphone of the assistive listening device to draw the child's

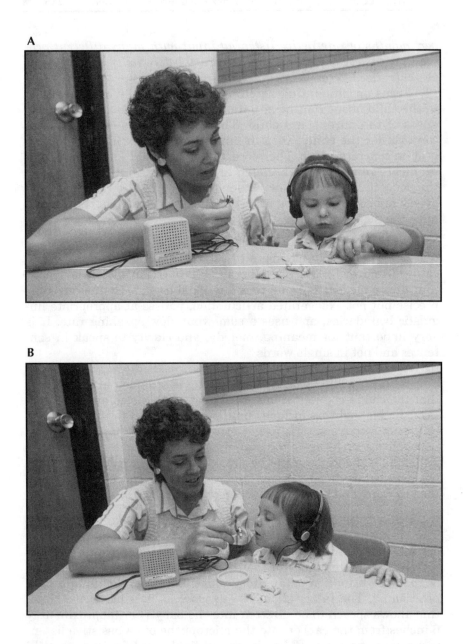

Figure 7–2. The microphone of a mild gain hard-wired unit is moved from the parent **(A)** to the child **(B)** to facilitate turntaking while enhancing the S/N ratio of both the parent's and child's speech.

attention to crucial word-sound differences; differences can be exaggerated to assist the child to hear distinctions among speech sounds. For example, a teacher might say, "Listen, Johnny, I said c-c-*cat*, not sss*sat*, Can you hear the difference?"

Parents should be instructed by the audiologist to listen to the child's personal FM system to determine if it is functioning properly. A second reason for listening to the system, especially if it has been provided by the school, is to determine whether the parents are satisfied with the signal their child is receiving. Some systems that are in perfect working order provide signals that are so poor that the child might as well not even bother to wear it. Do not accept the unit at face value. Listen to it. If it sounds bad (garbled, fuzzy, static, intermittent) to a person with normal hearing, imagine what it sounds like to a child who is hearing impaired. Remember, the young infant or child is *not* capable of telling adults that his or her equipment is not functioning properly; therefore, he or she may be forced to function for days, weeks, or months at a time with a poor signal *unless* the equipment is monitored daily.

TEACH THE CHILD TO LOCATE SOUNDS. If a child has had inconsistent, limited, or no experience with sound, he or she probably has learned to function in daily life using other sensory cues, usually visual, or cues dependent on the information he or she is able to detect. The young child may appear unresponsive to sound when, in reality, the unresponsiveness is directly tied to the lack of meaning that the sound conveys to him or her.

A crucial step in young children's aural habilitation is development of the ability to localize or find different sounds in their environments. Children who make no response to sounds that are known to be within their hearing range must actively be taught to find where the sound is coming from. As Lasky (1983) stated: "Processing information includes an awareness that a signal exists and a recognition that the signal carries meaning to be interpreted, comprehended, accepted or rejected, responded to, and perhaps remembered" (p. 11). Put another way by Edwards (1991), "a child's competency in listening develops not simply from having something to listen *to*, but also from something to listen *for*" (p. 389).

It is important to focus the infant or child's attention on meaningful sounds, both speech and environmental. Cue listening behaviors by saying the word "listen," and then pointing to your ear or to the child's ear (see Figure 7–3). For example, initially the

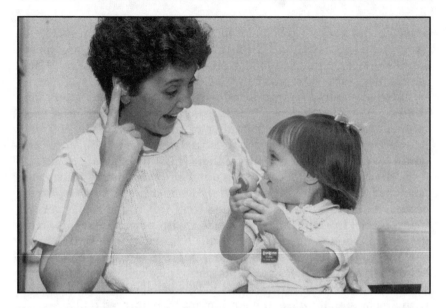

Figure 7–3. Cue listening and call attention to sounds by saying the word "listen" and pointing to your ear or the child's to emphasize auditory learning.

mother may stand behind the child with several different noise-makers that the parents know the child should be able to hear. Dad, or grandma, should casually occupy the child's attention (cued by the word "listen"). Mother presents the sound (rings the bell, squeaks the toy, hits the drum). If the child responds (localizes to the sound), liberal amounts of positive praise are in order (Good job! You heard that drum. What was that? Was that a bell? Wow! You heard that). These types of short sessions should be repeated frequently with different types of sounds and should progress to less formal measures once it is determined that the child will search. If no successful responses occur, the educational audiologist **must** be informed. Setting adjustments or repairs to the hearing aid may be needed. The possibility of a deterioration or fluctuation in hearing sensitivity also must be considered, especially in young children who may be prone to middle ear infections.

Parents also need to sharpen their own "incidental" listening skills because they may pick up on casual sounds to which the child should respond and which can be reinforced. Examples of these sounds are the telephone, a train whistle, car horn, doorbell, buzzers in dryers, or barking dogs. Acknowledge with positive reinforcement that the child responded to the sound.

Once the child knows what to listen "for," parents can start to attach meaning to different sounds that occur specifically in the child's own environment. The clinician should emphasize to the parent that their narrative about the sound is what makes it meaningful. A short list of common examples follows:

Sound	Response
doorbell	Oh listen, there's the doorbell. Someone's here. Who do you think it is? Lets go see. Or, Oh listen, there's the doorbell. Grandma's here! Hurry, let's go see her.
dryer buzzer	There's the buzzer. Did you hear that? Time to go get the clothes out of the dryer.
phone	Listen, do you hear the phone? Hello, who's there? Maybe it's daddy. Hi daddy. How are you?
dog bark	Listen, do you hear Skip? He's outside at the door. Quiet Skip. We're coming to let you in. Or Do you hear Skip? What do you think he wants? I bet he wants in/out, etc.

By helping the child search for sounds that are out of his or her visual field, the parent will help the child learn that objects and people make sounds and those sounds can be associated, in a predictable fashion, with the source (see Figure 7–4).

Parents and clinicians should use words and phrases that encourage and reinforce listening behaviors, for example: "I heard you"; "You heard that"; "You knew daddy was speaking"; "I like it when you listen"; "You looked at me when I called your name because you were listening"; "You heard me the very first time that I called, Wow!"

Naturally, the ultimate goal in developing the child's listening skills is to provide a basis for his or her language acquisition and the ability to comprehend what is heard. Once the child has begun to associate meaning and sounds (data input), language development begins to emerge. Children who are hearing impaired have the same capacity for learning language that children with normal hearing have (Brackett, 1997; Ross, Brackett, & Maxon, 1991); therefore, they should acquire speech patterns along the same developmental time lines as children with normal hearing (Ling, 1989) relative to their age of amplification.

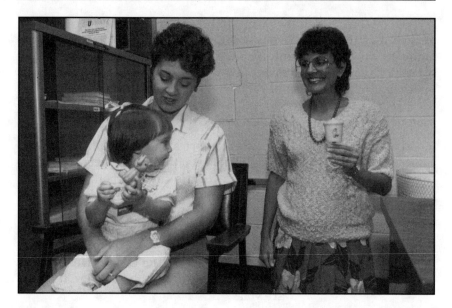

Figure 7–4. The accurate identification and localization of meaningful sounds with their source is another listening task.

Reading to the Child

Keeping in mind the acoustic filter effect of hearing impairment, begin reading to the child during his or her first year of life on a daily basis. Make sure that the books chosen are age-appropriate for the child. Very young children who have not yet developed competent listening skills and an adequate language base will have difficulty understanding stories that are beyond their level of comprehension. Books appropriate for young children are primarily picture books with limited text. An excellent source and starting point are Caldecott Medal books. This medal is awarded annually to the illustrator of the most distinguished American picture book. See Table 7–3 for a complete listing of these books.

Picture books allow the adult and the child to initiate conversation and vocabulary based on what he or she sees and is interested in. One of the best resources for the parent is the librarian in the children's department of the local library. These professionals are familiar with quality literature on a variety of topics for children. They have the ability to guide parents to books to help them to carry out a theme or supplement activities and experiences in which the child is involved. Many libraries also hold toddler story-

Table 7–3. The Caldecott Medal Books.

Year of Publication	Book Title	Author/Illustrator
1938	Animals of the Bible	Fish/Lathrop
1939	Mei Li	Hanforth
1940	Abraham Lincoln	D'Aulaire
1941	They Were Strong and Good	Lawson
1942	Make Way for Ducklings	McCloskey
1943	The Little House	Burton
1944	Many Moons	Thurber/Slobodkin
1945	Prayer for a Child	Field
1946	The Rooster Crows	Petersham
1947	The Little Island	MacDonald/Weisgard
1948	White Snow, Bright Snow	Tresselt/Duvoisin
1949	The Big Snow	Hader
1950	Song of the Swallows	Politi
1951	The Egg Tree	Milhous
1952	Finders Keepers	Will & Nicholas
1953	The Biggest Bear	Ward
1954	Madeline's Rescue	Bemelmans
1955	Cinderella	Perrault/Brown
1956	Frog Went A'courtin'	Langstaff Rojankovsky
1957	A Tree is Nice	Udry/Simont
1958	A Time of Wonder	McCloskey
1959	Chanticleer and the Fox	Cooney
1960	Nine Days to Christmas	Ets
1961	Baboushka and the Three Kings	Robbins/Sidjakov
1962	Once a Mouse	Brown
1963	The Snowy Day	Keats
1964	Where the Wild Things Are	Sendak
1965	May I Bring a Friend?	DeRegniers Montresor
1966	Always Room for One More	Nicleodhas Hogrogian
1967	Sam, Bangs & Moonshine	Ness
1968	Drummer Hoff	Emberly
1969	The Fool of The World and the Flying Ship	Ransome Shjulevita
1970	Sylvestor and the Magic Pebble	Steig
1971	A Story—A Story	Haley
1972	One Fine Day	Hogrogian
1973	The Funny Little Woman	Mosel/Lent
1974	Duffy and the Devil	Zemach

(continued)

Table 7–3. *(continued)*

Year of Publication	Book Title	Author/Illustrator
1975	Arrow to the Sun	McDermott
1976	Why Mosquitos Buzz in People's Ears	Aardema/Dillon
1977	Ahanti to Zulu: African Traditions	Musgrove/Dillan
1978	Noah's Ark	Revius/Spier
1979	The Girl Who Loved Wild Horses	Goble
1980	Ox-Cart Man	Hall/Cooney
1981	Fables	Lobel
1982	Jumanji	VanAllsburg
1983	Shadows	Brown
1984	The Glorious Flight	Provensen
1985	Saint George and the Dragon	Hodges/Hyman
1986	Polar Express	VanAllsburg
1987	Hey Al!	Vorinks/Egielski
1988	Owl Moon	Volen
1989	Song and Dance Man	Ackerman/Gammell
1990	Lon Po Po	Young
1991	Black and White	Macaulay
1992	Tuesday	Weisner
1993	Mirette on the High Wire	McCully
1994	Grandfather's Journey	Say
1995	Smoky Night	Bunting; illus. Dias
1996	Officer Buckle and Gloria	Rathmann
1997	Golem	Wiesniewski
1998	Rapunzel	Zelinsky

hour sessions that focus on the interests and developmental level of young children. The reader is referred to Cullinan (1992) and to Trelease (1995) for more information about how to read to young children.

■ FAMILY INTERACTION

The focus of intervention for the infant or young child is not on formal lessons but rather on optimizing all interactions, especially those that occur routinely throughout his or her daily life. Certain guidelines can be followed to provide the learning situation with a degree of structure and continuity, and especially with an auditory focus. The goal is the creation of a meaningful and ongoing "auditory world" for the child. Following are some points that can facilitate learning through family interactions:

1. *The family needs a conceptual framework in which common sense and thoughtful transactions can occur.* Strategies for making the child with hearing problems a full member of the family take place within an understanding of how hearing problems interfere with incidental learning. Because a child with a hearing problem has difficulty overhearing the conversations of others, she or he misses an enormous amount of information and social cues that typical children just "pick up." Therefore, the family needs to bring information directly to the child and inform the child of the topic under discussion. If the topic changes, the child should be told. If conversations between family members occur outside of the child's earshot, someone should tell the child about the content, or use the remote microphone of the FM system as a means of including the child. Family members need to talk about events, thinking processes, and feelings that they may not be in the habit of voicing. The child needs to be encouraged to "listen in" to the conversations of others.

2. Use an FM system at home to facilitate distance hearing and overhearing—to allow the child to "listen in" to conversations of family members, thereby gaining incidental information.

3. Focus on the *conversational interaction* between the parent and child, using *clear speech* and *acoustic highlighting.*

4. *Specific names (nouns)* of objects should be used to expand the child's vocabulary rather than referring to objects as "it," "them," "those," or "they."

5. Call attention to and teach *pragmatic skills* such as turn-taking, manners, and so on.

6. Use every opportunity to *emphasize prepositions* because, as unstressed parts of speech, they are difficult to hear. Prepositions are critical parts of speech for bridging concrete to abstract concepts. For example, a child needs to understand what it means to be "behind" someone in line before he or she can bridge to the more abstract meaning of being "behind" in one's taxes.

When more thoughtful activities are orchestrated by the family, the following guidelines can be helpful (Parents and Families of Natural Communication, Inc, 1998):

1. Plan one-on-one activities at a time of day that is usually quiet, calm, and unlikely to be disturbed by family commotion.
2. Activities should take place when the child is well rested and generally cooperative.
3. Adequate time should be allowed for completion of an activity without rushing to squeeze too much into a reduced time frame. It is better to thoroughly accomplish a small task than to attempt to do too much in too short a time.
4. Lessons can be skill-based, theme-based, or both. A *skill-based* approach focuses on the active teaching of specific skills selected from the list of goals that was formulated under the guidance of the child's therapist or teacher. Early on, these skills might involve learning colors, prepositions, 2- or 3-item sequencing, or phonics. A *theme-based* approach focuses on discussing a chosen topic and emphasizing the diversity of vocabulary and concept development it contains. Examples of themes include a trip to the circus or zoo, a seasonal change (weather), a holiday, family, baking, cowboys, or the solar system. Often, skills and themes are combined, for example pointing out the colors seen at a circus.

Four auditory skills development curricula that may be of interest to clinicians and parents are:

1. *The Auditory Skills Instructional Planning System.* There are five components to this system; one or all sections may be selected:

    Auditory Skills Curriculum

    Auditory Skills Curriculum—Preschool Supplement

    Test of Auditory Comprehension (TAC)

    Audio Worksheets

    Obtained from Foreworks, Box 82289, Portland, Oregon, 97282

    Phone (503) 653-2614

2. *Developmental Approach to Successful Listening II (DASL II).*

   Obtained from Resource Point, 61 Inverness Drive East, Suite 200, Englewood, CO 80112-9726

   Phone 1-800-688-8788

3. *Listening Games for Littles.* This includes listening ideas and listening tips in a developmental sequence for parents and professionals working with children ages 4 and under.

   Obtained from Word Play Publications, P.O. Box 8048, London, Ontario, Canada N6G 4X1

   Phone: 519-472-7762

4. *Speech Perception Instructional Curriculum Evaluation (SPICE).* This is a teacher-friendly auditory training curriculum designed for use with children who are hearing impaired, ages 3 years and up, with cochlear implants and/or hearing aids.

   Obtained from Central Institute for the Deaf, 818 South Euclid Ave., St. Louis, MO 63110

   Phone: 314-977-0000

■ CONCLUSIONS

The purpose of this book has been to provide information about hearing and listening as the cornerstones of early communication programming. Any infant or child who is at risk for developmental disabilities also is at risk for auditory disorders due to the strong association of hearing impairment with health measures.

Even a minimal, mild, or moderate hearing impairment, or a unilateral hearing impairment, or a fluctuating hearing impairment can sabotage communication and language development by diluting access to critical auditory centers of the brain. There is no such thing as an *insignificant* hearing impairment. Consequently, a child's hearing sensitivity must be known and accessed. The speech-to-noise ratio must be maximized for the reception of intelligible speech through the use of appropriate amplification and/or assistive technologies. Listening strategies must be employed to create an auditory-focused world and to teach the child to derive meaning from spoken communication.

The pediatric audiologist is the member of the early intervention team who can (a) provide knowledge of the auditory system; (b) interpret the detection of speech sounds through an understanding of acoustic phonetics; (c) furnish ongoing information about aided and unaided hearing sensitivity; (d) provide technological assistance in enhancing the speech-to-noise ratio through the use of hearing aids, assistive listening devices, and noise management procedures; and (e) supply suggestions for focusing on listening strategies as the basis for communicative interactions.

This book provided evidence that *hearing* is the most effective modality for teaching spoken language (speech), reading, and cognitive skills to infants and young children. With today's incredible amplification technology—as well as the opportunity for early identification and early intervention that is based on our knowledge of child development and the neural plasticity of auditory brain function—children with hearing loss, as well as typical children, have a world of options that were unavailable to them even 10 years ago. Because the purpose of early intervention is the enhancement of a child's functional outcome, maximizing a child's hearing with subsequent impact on brain development is a primary consideration.

■ APPENDIX 7A. TESTS OF AUDITORY SKILLS AND SPEECH PERCEPTION[1]

The Auditory Perception of Alphabet Letters Test (APAL) (1988)

AUTHORS: M. Ross and K. Randolph

TEST DESCRIPTION: The APAL test was developed for use with children who are hearing impaired, children for whom the commonly used WIPI, NU-CHIPS, and PBK tests are unsuitable.

The APAL test uses the oral production of the names of the letters of the alphabet as stimuli. The test incorporates a closed set response format of the 26 alphabet letters, which, although sizable, is among the first lists that are learned by children.

Live voice presentation should precede testing with audiotape. During actual testing for a score, the usefulness of the test will be diminished if an examiner uses live voice presentation. It is firmly believed that the recorded version is a crucial element in the clinical value of the APAL test. Five test forms are available. The first four stimuli in each list are used as practice items.

Scoring is weighted according to how close acoustically the response is to the correct answer.

The APAL test, incorporating the weighted error scoring scheme, offers a reliable and discriminating measure of the receptive capabilities of children who are hearing impaired.

DISTRIBUTED BY: Auditec of St. Louis, 2515 S. Big Bend Blvd., St. Louis, MO 63143. Telephone: (314) 781-8890

PRICE: Approximately $57.00 (includes an audiocassette recording of test)

Word Intelligibility by Picture Identification (WIPI) (1971)

AUTHORS: M. Ross and J. Lerman

TEST DESCRIPTION: WIPI is a word recognition test that utilizes six colored pictures per plate (closed set). The child points to the picture upon hearing the associated word.

---

[1]The author wishes to thank Donald Goldberg, Ph.D., Assistant Professor, College of Wooster, Ohio, for providing much of the information on the tests summarized in this appendix.

The WIPI was originally developed for young children who are hearing impaired.

It has four equivalent lists of 25 words each. The test has one practice plate. Each word should be preceded by a carrier phrase such as "show me." The child makes his or her choice by pointing to one of the pictures. A test assistant should tell the examiner the response the child selects (versus stating whether the answer is correct or incorrect). The test assistant should help maintain the child's attention and interest, as well as turn the pages of the test booklet after each choice by the child.

Testing can be completed auditorily, visually (speechreading), or in a combined (bimodal, audiovisual) condition.

DISTRIBUTED BY: Auditec of St. Louis, 2515 S. Big Bend Blvd, St. Louis, MO 63143. Telephone: (314) 781-8890

PRICE: Approximately $66.00 (includes test booklet and forms)
ALSO AVAILABLE: Audiocassette recording of test stimuli ($27.00)

Sound Effects Recognition Test (SERT) (1977)

AUTHORS: T. Finitzo-Hieber, N. Matkin, E. Cherow-Skalka, and I. Gerling

TEST DESCRIPTION: The authors state that every audiologic evaluation must include an assessment of auditory discrimination (recognition) ability, yet conventional monosyllabic speech measures are not always feasible for use with children due to oral language limitations. The SERT was therefore developed to measure sound effects recognition.

Gross environmental stimuli are utilized. Stimuli are presented via an audiocassette recording. The child is required to point to one of four pictures per picture plate (page). Presentation is at 25 to 40 dB SL (re: the SAT).

POPULATION: The SERT includes 30 items (3 equivalent 10-item subtests). The SERT reportedly is appropriate for children between the ages of 3;0 and 6;6 years.

INSTRUCTIONS: Look at all of the pictures, listen for the sound, and then point to the picture that goes with that sound.

DISTRIBUTED BY: Auditec of St. Louis, 2515 S. Big Bend Blvd., St. Louis, MO 63143. Telephone: (314) 781-8890

PRICE: Approximately $73.00 (includes tape, test manual, picture plates, and forms)

The Minimal Auditory Capabilities Battery (MAC Battery) (1981, 1985)

AUTHORS: E. Owens, D. Kellser, C. Telleeen, and E. Schubert (1981). The Minimal Auditory Capabilities (MAC) Battery. *Hearing Aid Journal*, *34*, 9, 32, 34; E. Owens, D. Kessler, M. Raggio, and E. Schubert (1985). Analysis and Revision of the Minimal Auditory Capabilities (MAC) Battery. *Ear and Hearing*, *6*(6), 280-290.

POPULATION: This is a test battery specifically developed to assess individuals who are profoundly, postlingually hearing impaired. The test can be used for hearing aid users and the assessment of potential cochlear implant candidates.

DESCRIPTION: The MAC includes 13 subtests and a speechreading assessment subtest. Subtests include the following:

1. Question/statement test
2. Vowel test
3. Spondee recognition test
4. Noise voice test
5. Accent test
6. *CID Everyday Sentences*
7. Initial consonant test
8. Spondee same/different test
9. Words in context (SPIN test)
10. Everyday sounds
11. Monosyllabic word test (NU #6)
12. Four-choice spondee test
13. Final consonant test

Plus visual enhancement: *CID Everyday Sentences*

A. *Without* amplification
B. *With* amplification

Test is on audiotape. Complete testing may take up to 2–3 hours.

AVAILABLE FROM: Auditec of St. Louis, 2515 S. Big Bend Blvd., St. Louis, MO 63143. Telephone: (314) 781-8890

PRICE: Approximately $90.50 (2 tapes, scoring, and response forms)

Glendonald Auditory Screening Procedure (GASP!) (1982)

AUTHOR: N. Erber, (1982). In *Auditory Training*. Washington, DC: Alexander Graham Bell Association for the Deaf.

TEST DESCRIPTION: This is an auditory procedure that evaluates the speech perception (listening) skills of a child who is hearing impaired via three subtests:

1. Phoneme detection
2. Word identification
3. Sentence comprehension

A child's performance is described not only on the basis of how many items he or she perceives correctly, but also on the basis of the number and type of adaptive strategies the teacher or clinician must apply to help the child succeed.

Phoneme Detection: A child is asked to respond *YES* (head nod) or point to the yes picture if he or she hears something, and *NO* (shake head) or point to the no picture if he or she hears nothing. Ten consonants and, periodically, a silent oral articulation are presented auditorily.

Word Identification: This subtest is administered to determine whether the child can identify words (in a limited set with only picture cues) on the basis of their spectral qualities or can only categorize them by their intensity patterns. A set of 12 words (nouns) are pictured, representative of four different stress-pattern categories: 3 monosyllabic words, 3 trochaic words, and 3 trisyllabic words. Child is asked to point to the words he or she hears. The stimuli are presented auditorily. Results are reported based on an exact word identification score and a categorization score based on the child's ability to correctly identify a word within the same stress pattern.

Sentence Comprehension (Question): Ten simple questions are provided and are asked without objects or principal prompts. (Most 6-year-old children who are hearing impaired can answer the question stimuli.)

Northwestern University Children's Perception of Speech (NU-CHIPS) (1980)

AUTHORS: L. Elliott and D. Katz

POPULATION: The NU-CHIPS test was developed as a speech discrimination (recognition) test for children and other persons having a language age as young as 3 years.

TEST DESCRIPTION: The test utilizes a closed set (four pictures per page). Some picture foils are phonemically similar to the test word. The test requires a picture-pointing response.

MATERIALS INCLUDE: Technical manual; four test forms (equivalent lists), each including the same monosyllabic nouns in a different randomization; audiotape recordings including a male and a female talker; two picture-response books; and answer sheets.

The NU-CHIPS test should be administered at 30-40 dB SL relative to the speech reception (recognition) threshold (SRT) or Fletcher Average (the average of thresholds obtained for the two best frequencies among 500, 1000, and 2000 Hz). A test assistant should tell the examiner the response the child selects (versus stating whether the answer is correct or incorrect). The test assistant should help maintain the child's attention and interest, as well as turn the page of the test booklet after each choice by the child.

Complete test: 50 items

Half-list: 25 words

DISTRIBUTED BY: Auditec of St. Louis, 2515 S. Big Bend Blvd., St. Louis, MO 63143. Telephone: (314) 781-8890

PRICE: Approximately $69.00

Early Speech Perception Test (ESP) (1990)

AUTHORS: J. Moog and A. Geers

POPULATION: The ESP test battery is designed for young children who are profoundly hearing impaired with limited vocabulary and language skills.

Colorful picture cards and, for younger children, interesting toys representing the words on the standard and low-verbal versions, are included in the complete ESP test kit. The words used in the ESP test are known by the majority of children who are hearing impaired, by the age of six, and can be identified by children who are not yet able to read.

The ESP test can be administered in 20 minutes or less. The test can be used with clients 3 years of age and older.

TEST DESCRIPTION: Standard Version Includes:

Pattern Perception Subtest

Word-Spondee Identification Subtest

Word-Monosyllabic Identification Subtest

Low-Verbal Version Includes:

Pattern Perception training

- "aaahhh" vs. "hop hop"
- trochees
- three syllable words

Pattern Perception Subtest

Word Identification Subtest (Spondees and Monosyllable Identification)

The ESP test allows for the categorization of children who are profoundly hearing impaired into one of four speech perception categories:

Category 1: no pattern perception

Category 2: pattern perception

Category 3: some word identification

Category 4: consistent word identification *and* defines in more detail their abilities within the category.

PUBLISHER: Central Institute for the Deaf, 818 South Euclid Ave., St. Louis, MO 63110. Telephone: (314) 977-0000

PRICE: Approximately $150.00 (includes manual, response forms, box of toys, full-color picture cards, and audiocassette)

ALSO AVAILABLE: Random access and audiotape (alternate randomization) stimuli prepared by G. Popelka and M. Russo.

Children's Auditory Test (CAT) (1976)

AUTHORS: N. Erber and Alencewicz, (1976). Audiologic Evaluation of Deaf Children. *Journal of Speech and Hearing Disorders,* *41*(2), 256–267.

TEST DESCRIPTION: This is an auditory assessment procedure that evaluates the speech perception skills of children who are hearing impaired. It makes use of 4 monosyllabic words, 4 trochees, and 4 spondees. All are pictorially represented.

The CAT enables the examiner to determine whether a child who is severely or profoundly hearing impaired can make use of spectral cues and demonstrate exact word identification abilities and/or use suprasegmental cues in the identification of stress patterns only.

A percent correct score based on word identification, and a percent correct score based on identification of syllabic categories or stress patterns are reported. Testing is completed auditorily.

Monosyllables	Trochees	Spondees
bed	button	airplane
cat	chicken	baseball
duck	doctor	popcorn
pig	turtle	toothbrush

Auditory Numbers Test (ANT) (1980)

AUTHOR: N. Erber, (1980). Use of the Auditory Numbers Test to Evaluate Speech Perception Abilities of Children Who are Hearing Impaired. *Journal of Speech and Hearing Disorders*, 45(4), 527–532.

DESCRIPTION: ANT is an auditory assessment procedure that evaluates the speech perception skills of children who are hearing impaired. It assists in the determination of whether a young child can perceive spectral aspects of speech or only gross temporal acoustic patterns.

ANT makes use of pictures that depict a varied number of ants (1–5).

Following training, the testing evaluates whether the child can identify the cues 1,2,3,4, and 5 or only the stress patterns 1; 1,2; 1,2,3; 1,2,3,4; and 1,2,3,4,5. Testing is completed auditorily.

Test of Auditory Comprehension (TAC) (1981)

AUTHOR: J. Trammell

DESCRIPTION: The TAC is a comprehensive test instrument developed for individual use with pupils who are hearing impaired. It assesses auditory functioning in the areas of discrimination, memory-sequence, and figure-ground.

Results of the TAC Provide:

1. A measure of a variety of skills inherent in the auditory processing of speech.
2. A basis for selection of appropriate auditory skill objectives.
3. An evaluation of growth in the acquisition of auditory abilities.
4. An indicator for educational placement decisions.

Total T scores, and T scores for each subtest are calculated.

Norms: Available for ages 4–17 years.

Norms are available based on PTA; delineating subjects with moderate, moderately-severe, severe, and profound hearing impairments.

Components: Screening task (samples subtests 2–6)

Subtest 1: Linguistic vs. Non-linguistic
Subtest 2: Linguistic/Human
Non-linguistic/Environmental
Subtest 3: Stereotypic Messages
Subtest 4: Single Element, Core Noun Vocabulary
Subtest 5: Recalls Two Critical Elements
Subtest 6: Recalls Four Critical Elements
Subtest 7: Sequences Three Events
Subtest 8: Recalls Five Details
Subtest 9: Sequences Three Events With Competing Messages
Subtest 10: Recalls Five Details With Competing Messages

RELATIONSHIP OF SUBTEST CONTENT TO CURRICULUM AREAS TAC SUBTESTS

Auditory Skills Curriculum area	1	2	3	4	5	6	7	8	9	10
Discrimination										
Suprasegmental	x	x	x			x	x	x	x	x
Segmental			x	x	x	x	x	x	x	x
Memory Sequencing										
Recall elements					x	x	x	x	x	x
Sequence events						x	x	x	x	x
Auditory Cognitive										
Story comprehension							x	x	x	x
Figure-Ground										
Verbal Distraction									x	x

Test stimuli are on audio cassette, to be delivered at 56 dB HL.

PUBLISHER: Foreworks Publications, Box 82289, Portland, Oregon 97282. Telephone: (503) 653-2614

PRICE: Approximately $90.00

ALSO AVAILABLE: Audio Worksheets

Phonetic Level Evaluation (PLE) (1976)

AUTHOR: D. Ling (1976). *In Speech for the Hearing Impaired Child: Theory and Practice.* Washington, DC: Alexander Graham Bell Association for the Deaf

TEST DESCRIPTION: PLE is a speech production evaluation procedure to be used in conjunction with Ling's text on training speech to children who are hearing impaired. It evaluates both nonsegmental and segmental aspects of speech, including spontaneous vocalization and vocalization on demand, vocal duration, vocal intensity, vocal pitch, vowels and diphthongs, simple consonants, and blends.

Targets are elicited by imitation of the examiner. Responses are classified as being produced consistently (✓), inconsistently (+), or not at all (−). The primary purpose of the PLE is to provide the teacher or clinician with clearly defined teaching goals.

The SKI*HI Language Development Scale (LDS) (1979)

AUTHORS: S. Tonelson and S. Watkins

POPULATION: For children who are hearing impaired: Infancy to 5 years of age.

PURPOSE: The objective of the LDS is to assess the receptive and expressive language skills of the child who is hearing impaired, and to determine the child's current level of functioning as compared to norm referenced development scales.

TEST DESCRIPTION: The LDS makes use of lists of expressive and receptive language skills. The lists are divided into units that are representative of a specific age range.

The LDS does not emphasize auditory items and most such items have been eliminated from the receptive scale. It does not penalize children using total communication; credit is given to the understanding and use of signs. The LDS is administered through parent observation of their child's language skills. The parent is trained and advised regarding the test administration by a parent trainer (the clinician).

The LDS is given to the parent to take home for a 1-week period in which time they will evaluate their child's communication skills by looking for the items in the list that the parent advisor had selected.

The LDS is scored with pluses (+) and minuses (−). A 50% criteria is required for both the receptive and expressive portions in order to be considered to be functioning in that unit (age range).

PUBLISHER: Hope, Inc., 55 East 100 North, Suite 203, Logan, Utah 84321. Telephone: (435) 752-9533.

PRICE: Approximately $.95 each for 1–50 forms; $5.90 for instruction book.

Developmental Activities Screening Inventory II (DASI-II) (1984)

AUTHORS: R. Fewell and M. B. Langley

POPULATION: Children functioning between the ages of birth to 60 months, although the lowest scorable age is 1 month.

TEST PURPOSE/OBJECTIVE: Designed as an informal developmental screening measure for children functioning between the ages of birth and 60 months.

DESCRIPTION: An individually administered nonverbal test. The 67 test items in 11 developmental levels tap a variety of skills, including fine-motor coordination, cause-effect and means-end relationships, association, number concepts, size determination, memory, spatial relationships, object function, and seriation. These skills represent behaviors frequently included in tests of early development.

Begin administering test items one level below examiner's estimate of the child's developmental age.

Basal—passes all items in a level

Ceiling—fails all items at one level

PERCEPTUAL/CONCEPTUAL COMPONENTS: (appendix includes an item analysis for DASI-II items):

Sensory Intactness   Construction Objects in Space

Sensorimotor Organization   Memory

Causality   Visual Pursuit-Object Permanence

Imitation   Means-end Relationship

Discrimination   Association

Quantitative Reasoning   Seriation

Spatial Relationships   Reasoning

Behaviors relating to Objects

TESTING TIME: Variable. Often 25 to 30 minutes

SCORING: Child receives one raw score point for each item that is passed (credit is also given for each item below the level where the child passed all six items.) Total number of raw score points is converted into a developmental age (DA) (in months). A developmental quotient (DQ) is computed using the following formula: $DQ = DA/CA \times 100$.

SCORE INTERPRETATION GUIDE:

> 140 Superior

121 to 140 Above Average

80 to 120 Average

60 to 79 Below Average

< 60 Poor

NOTES: For every skill (67) tapped in the DASI-II; instructional suggestions/activities are provided for its development and refinement (42 pages worth).

Some materials are included for the test. A variety of additional materials must be obtained.

VALIDITY: Concurrent validity established. DASI-II was demonstrated to *not* penalize children with known language deficits.

PUBLISHER: PRO-ED, 8700 Shoal Creek Blvd, Austin, TX 78757-6897. Telephone: (512) 451-3246

PRICE: Approximately $79.00

Preschool Language Scale—3 (PLS–3) (1992)

AUTHORS: I. Zimmerman, V. Steiner, and R. Pond

TEST PURPOSE/OBJECTIVES: The PLS–3 provides a survey of an infant or child's early language comprehension and use. It was designed to be a diagnostic and screening instrument capable of systematically appraising the early stages of language development.

TEST DESCRIPTION: Tasks are arranged into two subscales: Auditory Comprehension (which measures receptive skills) and Expressive Communication (which measures expressive skills). Both receptive and expressive language and prelanguage skills are measured in attention, vocal development, social communication, semantics, structure, and integrative thinking skills. PLS–3 now measures preverbal skills.

POPULATION: Norms available for infants and children, birth to 6 years of age.

TESTING TIME: Variable (approximately 30 minutes).

SCORING: Provides norm-referenced scores, including means and standard deviations by age group for children birth through 6 years. PLS–3 also can be used as a criterion-referenced test for older children who are functioning within the range of behaviors assessed by PLS–3; the test thus can evaluate what the child can do, and not just what they cannot do.

PUBLISHER: The Psychological Corporation, Order Service Center, P.O. Box 839954, San Antonio, TX 78283-3954. Telephone: (800) 228-0752. (800) 211-8378 Direct information and order line.

PRICE: $126.50

Test of Auditory Comprehension of Language— Revised (TACL-R) (1985)

AUTHORS: E. Carrow-Woolfolk

TEST PURPOSE/OBJECTIVE: The TACL-R provides an inventory of grammatical forms for observing a child's auditory comprehension behavior. The test helps to identify individuals who have receptive language disorders. It helps to guide the clinician towards specific areas of grammar that need additional testing and provides a means of measuring change in grammatical comprehension.

TEST DESCRIPTION: Individually administered. The TACL-R consists of 120 items presented in three sections of 40 items each in the areas of word classes and relations, grammatical morphemes, and elaborated sentences.

Each stimulus item is composed of a word or sentence and a corresponding plate that has three black-and-white line drawings. One of the three pictures for each item illustrates the meaning of the word, morpheme, or syntactic structure being tested. The examiner reads the stimulus aloud, and the subject is directed to point to the picture that he or she believes best represents the meaning of the word, phrase, or sentence spoken by the examiner. No oral response is required on the part of the subject.

Recommended starting points (based on chronological age) are provided.

POPULATION: Norms available for children 3;0 through 9;11.

TESTING TIME: Approximately 10 minutes.

SCORING: Basal and ceiling rules are provided for each section. Raw scored can be converted to percentile ranks, standard scores, standard error of measurement, age equivalents, and grade level scores.

RELIABILITY/VALIDITY: High internal consistency (split-half) and test-retest reliability. Content, construct, and criterion-related validity established.

PUBLISHER: Riverside Publishing Co., 425 Spring Lake Drive, Itasca, IL 60143. Telephone: (800) 323-9540

PRICE: Approximately $194.00

Boehm Test of Basic Concepts—Preschool Version (1986)

AUTHOR: A. Boehm

TEST PURPOSE/OBJECTIVES: Designed to measure a child's knowledge of 26 basic relational concepts considered necessary for achievement in the beginning of school.

TEST DESCRIPTION: Individually administered. Includes 5 warm-up items followed by 52 test questions (two items per concept). For each item, the examiner shows the child a picture and asks questions about it. Child responds by pointing to an appropriate portion of the picture.

CONCEPTS:

another	all	around	full
nearest	lowest	up	middle
across	both	largest	outside
missing	highest	down	under
tallest	after	backwards	shortest
many	together	smallest	before
finished	farthest		

POPULATION: Children 3 to 5 years of age (and older who have special educational needs).

TESTING TIME: Approximately 15 minutes.

SCORING: Scores for the pair of items that measure each concept are tallied—concept scores are therefore noted. Score on the total 52 individual items is then tallied for a total score.

Percentile scores and T-scores are provided. A table, "percentile equivalents of total scores by age" (with 5 age groupings) is available.

NOTE: A national standardization of Boehm-Preschool was completed.

RELIABILITY/VALIDITY: High internal consistency and test-retest reliability. Content and concurrent validity established.

PUBLISHER: The Psychological Corporation, Harcourt, Brace, Jovanovich, Inc., 555 Academic Court, San Antonio, TX 78204. Telephone: (800) 228-0752. (800) 211-8378 Direct information and order line.

PRICE: Approximately $114.50

Peabody Picture Vocabulary Test—Revised (RPVT-3) (1997)

AUTHORS: L. Dunn and L. Dunn

TEST PURPOSE/OBJECTIVE: Designed to measure a subject's (*hearing*) vocabulary for standard American English.

TEST DESCRIPTION: Individually administered. Two forms (A–B). For each item the examiner shows the subject a picture plate (four pictures per plate) and, for example, prompts, "show me _____." Subject responds by pointing to one picture. Includes five training plates. Total 175 test items possible.

POPULATION: Norms available for persons 2;6 through 40;11.

TESTING TIME: Approximately 15 to 20 minutes.

SCORING:

ᵓasal—8 consecutive correct responses.

Ceiling—8 consecutive responses containing 6 errors.

Recommended starting points (based on chronological age) are provided.

The raw score can be converted to a standard score equivalent; percentile rank; stanine; and age equivalent.

NOTE: A representative national standardization for the PPVT-R was completed.

RELIABILITY/VALIDITY: High internal consistency and alternate-forms reliability. Content and construct validity established.

PUBLISHER: American Guidance Service, P.O. Box 99, Circle Pines, MN 55014-1796. Telephone: (800) 328-2560

PRICE: Approximately $119.95

Structured Photographic Expressive Language Test— Preschool (SPELT-Preschool) (1983)

AUTHORS: E. Werner and J. Kresheck

TEST PURPOSE/OBJECTIVE: Designed to be a screening instrument to allow the examiner to identify children who may have difficulty in their expression of early developing morphological and syntactical features.

TEST DESCRIPTION: Individually administered. The visual stimuli are full color photographs of children engaged in childhood activities and of animals and objects. An item may have one or two photographs. The auditory stimuli are questions or statements said by the examiner. The examiner asks the questions or says the statement and presents the accompanying photograph(s) to the child. The child responds. Some of the items utilize a "close" technique. The examiner says an unfinished sentence to the child while presenting the photograph(s). The child completes the sentence supplying the missing form. The examiner writes down the subject's response.

STRUCTURES (25):

plural nouns	possessive nouns
personal pronouns	prepositions
auxiliary verbs	copulas

present and past tense of the main verbs

POPULATION: Children 3;0 through 5;11.

TESTING TIME: Approximately 3 to 10 minutes

SCORING: If the child's total raw score falls at or below the cutoff score for his or her age group (6 months intervals), further assessment is warranted. Percentiles for the different age groups are provided. Percents at which 3-, 4-, and 5-year-olds pass each test item are also provided.

The SPELT-Preschool includes a system of alternate response structures for assessment of Black English speakers.

RELIABILITY/VALIDITY: High test-retest, internal consistency, and interscorer reliability. Content, concurrent, and construct validity established.

PUBLISHER: Janelle Publications, Inc., P.O. Box 811, DeKalb, IL 60115. Telephone: (815) 756-2300 or (800) 888-8834.

PRICE: Approximately $79.00

■ APPENDIX 7B. INFORMATION ABOUT THE AUDITORY-VERBAL PHILOSOPHY

The following document, reprinted with permission of AVI from *The Auricle, 3,* 1991, was prepared by the Board of Directors of Auditory-Verbal International (AVI), and adopted as the official position statement of AVI in October of 1991. Members of the Board of Directors responsible for the development of the document include Nancy Caleffe-Schenck, Marian Ernst, Warren Estabrooks, Carol Flexer, Donald Goldberg, Chester Homer III, Daniel Ling, Judith Marlowe, Dennis Pappas, Doreen Pollack, Susann Schmid-Giovannini, Judy Simser, Sally Tannenbaum, Maxine Turnbull, and James Watson.

Auditory-Verbal

The Auditory-Verbal philosophy is a logical and critical set of guiding principles. These principles outline the essential requirements needed to realize the expectation that young children with hearing impairment can be educated to use even minimal amounts of amplified residual hearing. Use of amplified residual hearing in turn permits children with hearing impairment to learn to listen, to process verbal language, and to speak.

The goal of Auditory-Verbal practice is that children with hearing impairment can grow up in regular learning and living environments that enable them to become independent, participating, and contributing citizens in mainstream society. The Auditory-Verbal philosophy supports the basic human right that children with all degrees of hearing impairment deserve an opportunity to develop the ability to listen and to use verbal communication within their own family and community constellations.

The System of Principles of Auditory-Verbal Practice[1] are:

1. Supporting and promoting programs for the early detection and identification of hearing impairment and the auditory management of infants, toddlers and children so identified;

2. providing the earliest and most appropriate use of medical and amplification technology to achieve the maximum benefits available;

3. instructing primary caregivers in ways to provide maximal acoustic stimulation within meaningful contexts, and supporting the development of the most

---

[1]Principles of Auditory-Verbal Practice have been adapted from Pollack (1970, 1985).

favorable auditory learning environments for the acquisiton of spoken language;

4. seeking to integrate listening into the child's total personality in response to the environment;

5. supporting the view that communication is a social act, and seeking to improve spoken communicative interaction within the typical social dyad of infant/child with hearing impairment and primary caregiver(s), including the use of the parents as primary models for spoken language development, and implementing one-to-one teaching;

6. seeking to establish the child's integrated auditory system for the self-monitoring of emerging speech;

7. using natural sequential patterns of auditory, perceptual, linguistic and cognitive stimulation to encourage the emergence of listening, speech and language abilities;

8. making ongoing evaluation and prognosis of the development of listening skills an integral part of the (re)habilitative process;

9. and supporting the concepts of mainstreaming and integration of children with hearing impairment into regular education classes with appropriate support services and to the fullest extent possible.

Existing Evidence That Supports the Rationale for Auditory-Verbal Practice

1. The majority of children with hearing impairment have useful residual hearing; a fact known for decades (Bezold & Siebenmann, 1908; Goldstein, 1939; Urbantschitsch, 1982).

2. When properly aided, children with hearing impairment can detect most if not all of the speech spectrum (Beebe, 1953; Goldstein, 1939; Johnson, 1975, 1976; Ling, 1989; Ling & Ling, 1978; Pollack, 1970, 1985; Ross & Calvert, 1984).

3. Once ALL available residual hearing is accessed through amplification technology (e.g., binaural hearing aids and acoustically tuned earmolds, FM units, cochlear implants) in order to provide maximum detection of the speech spectrum, then a child will have the opportunity to develop language in a natural way through the auditory modality. That is, a

child with hearing loss need not automatically be a visual learner. Hearing, rather than being a passive modality that receives information, can be the active agent of cognitive development (Boothroyd, 1982; Goldberg & Lebahn, 1990; Robertson & Flexer, 1993; Ross & Calvert, 1984).

4. In order to benefit from the "critical periods" of neurological and linguistic development, then the identification of hearing impairment, use of appropriate amplification and medical technology, and stimulation of hearing must occur as early as possible (Clopton & Winfield, 1976; Johnson & Newport, 1989; Lennenberg, 1967; Marler, 1970; Newport, 1990).

5. If hearing is not accessed during the critical language learning years, a child's ability to use acoustic input meaningfully will deteriorate due to physiological (retrograde deterioration of auditory pathways), and psychosocial (attention, practice, learning) factors (Evans, Webster, & Cullen, 1983; Merzenich & Kaas, 1982; Patchett, 1977; Robertson & Irvine, 1989; Webster, 1983).

6. Current information about normal language development provides the framework and justification for the structure of Auditory-Verbal practice. That is, infants/toddlers/children learn language most efficiently through consistent and continual meaningful interactions in a supportive environment with significant caretakers (Kretschmer & Kretschmer, 1978; Lennenberg, 1967; Leonard, 1991; Ling, 1989; MacDonald & Gillette, 1989; Menyuk, 1977; Ross, 1990).

7. As verbal language develops through the auditory input of information, reading skills can also develop (Geers & Moog, 1989; Ling, 1989; Robertson & Flexer, 1993).

8. Parents in Auditory-Verbal programs do not have to learn sign language or cued speech. More than ninety percent of parents of children with hearing impairment have normal hearing (Moores, 1987). Studies show that over 90% of parents with normal hearing do not learn sign language beyond a basic preschool level of competency (Luetke-Stahlman & Moeller, 1987). Auditory-Verbal practice requires that care-

givers interact with a child through spoken language and create a listening environment which helps a child to learn.

9. If a severe or profound hearing loss automatically makes an individual neurologically and functionally "different" from people with normal hearing (Furth, 1964; Myklebust & Brutton, 1953), then the Auditory-Verbal philosophy would not be tenable. The fact is, however, that outcome studies show that individuals who have, since early childhood, been taught through the active use of amplified residual hearing, are indeed independent, speaking, and contributing members of mainstream society (Goldberg & Flexer, 1993; Ling, 1989; Yoshinaga-Itano & Pollack, 1988).

References

American Academy of Audiology. (1992). Say what . . . ? An introduction to hearing loss. [Audio tape].

American Academy of Audiology. (1997). Audiology: Scope of practice. *Audiology Today, 9*, 12–13.

American Speech-Language-Hearing Association. (1990a). Guidelines for audiometric symbols. *Asha, 32*(Suppl. 2), 25–30.

American Speech-Language-Hearing Association. (1990b). Guidelines for screening hearing impairments and middle ear disorders. *Asha, 32*(Suppl. 2), 17–24.

American Speech-Language-Hearing Association. (1991a). Amplification as a remediation technique for children with normal peripheral hearing. *Asha, 33*(Suppl. 3), 22–24.

American Speech-Language-Hearing Association. (1991b). Chronic communicable diseases and risk management in the schools. *Language, Speech, and Hearing Services in Schools, 22*, 345–352.

American Speech-Language-Hearing Association. (1991c). Joint Committee on Infant Hearing 1990 position statement. *Asha, 33*(Suppl. 5), 3–6.

American Speech-Language-Hearing Association. (1993). Guidelines for audiologic services in the schools. *Asha, 35*(Suppl. 10), 24–32.

American Speech-Language-Hearing Association. (1995). Position statement and guidelines for acoustics in educational settings. *Asha, 37*(Suppl. 14), 15–19.

Anderson, K. L. (1991). Hearing conservation in the public schools revisited. In C. Flexer (Ed.), Current audiologic issues in the educational management of children with hearing loss. *Seminars in Hearing, 12*, 340–364.

Audiologic screening of newborn infants who are at-risk for hearing impairment. (1989). *Asha, 31*, 89–92.

Auditory skills instructional planning system. (1986). Portland, OR: Foreworks.

Baker, R. C. (1991). Pitfalls in diagnosing acute otitis media. *Pediatric Annals, 20*, 591–598.

Balkany, T. J., Mischke, R. E., Downs, M. P., & Jafek, B. W. (1979). Ossicular abnormalities in Down's syndrome. *Otolaryngology—Head and Neck Surgery, 87*, 372–384.

Beebe, H. (1953). *A guide to help the severely hard of hearing child.* Basel/New York: Karger.

Bench, J., Hoffman, E., & Wilson, I. (1974). A comparison of live and video-record viewing of infant behavior under sound stimulation. I. Neonates. *Developmental Psychology, 7*, 455–464.

Bentler, R. A. (1996). What to look for in a hearing aid evaluation. In C. Flexer, D. Wray, R. Levitt, & R. Flexer, (Eds.), *How the student with hearing loss can succeed in college: A handbook for students, families, and professionals* (2nd ed., pp. 51–60). Washington, DC: The Alexander Graham Bell Association for the Deaf.

Berg, F. S. (1986). Characteristics of the target population. In F. S. Berg, J. C. Blair, J. H. Viehweg, & A. Wilson-Vlotman (Eds.), *Educational audiology for the hard of hearing child* (pp. 1–24). New York: Grune & Stratton.

Berg, F. S. (1987). *Facilitating classroom listening: A handbook for teachers of normal and hard of hearing students.* Boston: College-Hill Press/Little Brown.

Berg, F. S. (1993). *Acoustics and sound systems in schools.* San Diego: Singular Publishing Group.

Berg, F. S., Blair, J. C., & Benson, P. V. (1996). Classroom acoustics: The problem, impact, and solution. *Language, Speech, and Hearing Services in Schools, 27*, 16–20.

Berg, F. S., Blair, J. C., Viehweg, J. H., & Wilson-Vlotman, A. (Eds.). (1986). *Educational audiology for the hard of hearing child.* New York: Grune & Stratton.

Berlin, C. I. (Ed.). (1998). *Otoacoustic emissions: Basic science and clinical applications.* San Diego, CA: Singular Publishing Group.

Berlin, C. I., & Hood, L. J. (1987). Auditory brainstem response and middle ear assessment in children. In F. N. Martin (Ed.), *Hearing disorders in children* (pp. 151–184). Austin, TX: Pro-Ed.

Berman, S. A., Balkany, T. J., & Simmons, M. A. (1978). Otitis media in the neonatal intensive care unit. *Pediatrics, 62*, 198–201.

Bess, F. H. (1985). The minimally hearing-impaired child. *Ear and Hearing, 6*, 43–47.

Bess, F. H. (Ed.). (1988). *Hearing impairment in children.* Parkton, MD: York Press.

Bess, F. H., Gravel, J. S., & Tharpe, A. M. (Eds.). (1996). *Amplification for children with auditory deficits.* Nashville, TN: Bill Wilkerson Center Press.

Bess, F. H., Klee, T., & Culbertson, J. L. (1986). Identification, assessment and management of children with unilateral sensorineural hearing loss. *Ear and Hearing, 7*, 43–51.

Bess, F. H., Peek, B., & Chapman, J. (1979). Further observations on noise levels in infant incubators. *Pediatrics, 63,* 100.

Bezold, F. R., & Siebenmann, F. R. (1908). *Textbook of otology for physicians and students.* Chicago: E. H. Colegrove.

Blair, J. C.. (1986). Services needed. In F. S. Berg, J. C. Blair, S. H. Viehweg, & A. Wilson-Vlotman (Eds.), *Educational audiology for the hard of hearing child* (pp. 25–35). New York: Grune & Stratton.

Blair, J., Myrup, C., & Viehweg, S. (1989). Comparison of the effectiveness of hard-of-hearing children using three types of amplification. *Educational Audiology Monograph, 1,* 48–55.

Blake, R., Field, B., Foster, C., Platt, F., & Wertz, P. (1991). Effect of FM auditory trainers on attending behaviors of learning disabled children. *Language, Speech, and Hearing Services in Schools, 22,* 111–114.

Bluestone, C. D., Klein, J. O., Paradise, J. L., Eichenwald, H., Bess, F. H., Downs, M. P., Green, M., Berko-Gleason, J., Ventry, I. M., Gray, S. W., McWilliams, B. J., & Gates, G. A. (1983). Workshop on effects of otitis media on the child. *Pediatrics, 71,* 639–652.

Boothroyd, A. (1978). Speech perception and severe hearing loss. In M. Ross & T. G. Giolas (Eds.), *Auditory management of hearing-impaired children* (pp. 117–144). Baltimore: University Park Press.

Boothroyd, A. (1982). *Hearing impairments in young children.* Englewood Cliffs, NJ: Prentice-Hall.

Boothroyd, A. (1984). Getting the most out of hearing. The audiological and auditory management of hearing-impaired children. *Audiology, 9,* 15–26.

Boothroyd, A. (1997). Auditory development of the hearing child. *Scandinavian Audiology, 26(*Suppl. 46), 9–16.

Boothroyd, A., Geers, A. E., & Moog, J. S. (1991). Practical implications of cochlear implants in children. In S. Staller (Ed.), Multichannel cochlear implants in children [Special issue]. *Ear and Hearing, 12*(4, Suppl.), 81S–89S.

Boutte, V. (1998). A new age for advocacy. *Volta Voices, 5,* 19–21.

Brackett, D. (1997). Intervention for children with hearing impairment in general education settings. *Language, Speech and Hearing Services in Schools, 28,* 355–261.

Brackett, D., & Maxon, A. B. (1986). Device alternatives for the mainstreamed hearing-impaired child. *Language, Speech and Hearing Services in Schools, 17,* 115–125.

Brownell, W. E. (1990). Outer hair cell electromotility and otoacoustic emissions. *Ear and Hearing, 11,* 89–92.

Bryant, P. E., Bradley, L., MacLean, M., & Crossland, J. (1989). Nursery rhymes, phonological skills and reading. *Journal of Child Language, 16,* 407–428.

Busenbark, L., & Jenison, V. (1986). Assessing hearing aid function by listening check. *The Volta Review, 88,* 263–268.

Cargill S., & Flexer, C. (1989). Issues in fitting FM units to children with unilateral hearing losses: Two case studies. *Educational Audiology Monograph, 1,* 30–47.

Cargill S., & Flexer, C. (1991). Strategies for fitting FM units to children with unilateral hearing losses. *Hearing Instruments, 42*(7), 26–27.

Chermak, G. D., Curtis, L., & Seikel, J. A. (1996). The effectiveness of an interactive hearing conservation program for elementary school children. *Language, Speech, and Hearing Services in Schools, 27,* 29–34.

Chermak, G. D., & Musiek, F. E. (1997). *Central auditory processing disorders: New perspectives.* San Diego, CA: Singular Publishing Group.

Clark, G. M., Cowan, R. S. C., & Dowell, R. C. (1997). *Cochlear implantation for infants and children: Advances.* San Diego, CA: Singular Publishing Group.

Clark, J. G., & Martin, F. N. (1994). *Effective counseling in audiology: Perspectives and practice.* Englewood Cliffs, NJ: Prentice-Hall.

Clark, M. (1989). *Language through living for hearing-impaired children.* London: Hodder and Stoughton.

Clopton, B., & Winfield, J. A. (1976). Effect of early exposure to patterned sound on unit activity in rat inferior colliculus. *Journal of Neurophysiology, 39,* 1081–1089.

Code of Federal Regulations on Education. (1986). Title 34 Education (Parts 300–399). Washington, DC: Government Printing Office.

Cole, E., & Gregory, H. (Eds.). (1986). Auditory learning. *The Volta Review, 88,* 1–122.

Collins, S. H. (1989). *Sound hearing or . . . hearing what you miss.* [Audio tape]. Eugene, OR: Garlic Press.

Compton, C. L. (1991). *Doorways to independence.* [Videotape and book]. Washington, DC: Gallaudet University. (Available from Academy of Dispensing Audiologists, Columbia, SC. Telephone: [800] 445-8629)

Compton, C. L. (1993). Assistive technology for deaf and hard-of-hearing people. In J. Alpiner & P. McCarthy (Eds.), *Rehabilitative audiology: Children and adults* (2nd ed., pp. 441–468). Baltimore, MD: Williams & Wilkins.

Conway, L. C. (1990). Issues relating to classroom management. In M. Ross (Ed.), *Hearing-impaired children in the mainstream.* Parkton, MD: York Press.

Coplan, J. (1987). Deafness: Ever heard of it? Delayed recognition of permanent hearing loss. *Pediatrics, 79,* 206–213.

Cotton, R. T. (1991). The surgical management of chronic otitis media with effusion. *Pediatric Annals, 20,* 628–637.

Cox, L. C., & MacDonald, C. B. (1996). Large vestibular acqueduct syndrome: A tutorial and three case studies. *Journal of the American Academy of Audiology, 7,* 71–76.

Crandell, C. (1996). Effects of sound field FM amplificcation on the speech perception of ESL children. *Educational Audiology Monograph, 4,* 1–5.

Crandell, C. C., & Roeser, R. J. (1993). Incidence of excessive/impacted cerumen in individuals with mental retardation: A longitudinal investigation. *American Journal on Mental Retardation, 97*(5), 568–574.

Crandell, C. C., & Smaldino, J. J. (1996). Speech perception in noise by children for whom English is a second language. *American Journal of Audiology, 5,* 47–51.

Crandell, C., Smaldino, J., & Flexer, C. (1995). *Sound-field FM amplification: Theory and practical applications.* San Diego, CA: Singular Publishing Group.

Crandell, C. C., Smaldino, J. J., & Flexer, C. (1997). A suggested protocol for implementing sound-field FM technology in the educational setting. *Educational Audiology Monograph, 5*, 13–21.

Cranford, J. L., Thompson, N., Hoyer, E., & Faires, W. (1997). Brief tone discrimination by children with histories of early otitis media. *Journal of the American Academy of Audiology, 8*, 137–141.

Culbertson, J. L., & Gilbert, L. E. (1986). Children with unilateral sensorineural hearing loss: Cognitive, academic and social development. *Ear and Hearing, 7*, 38–42.

Cullinan, B. (1992). *Read to me: Raising kids who love to read.* New York: Scholastic.

Dahle, A. J., & McCollister, F. P. (1986). Hearing and otologic disorders in children with Down syndrome. *American Journal of Mental Deficiency, 90*, 636–642.

Davis, H., & Silverman, S. R. (1978). *Hearing and deafness* (4th ed.). New York: Holt, Rinehart and Winston.

Davis, J. (Ed.). (1990). *Our forgotten children: Hard-of-hearing pupils in the schools.* Bethesda, MD: Self Help for Hard of Hearing People.

Decker, T. N. (Ed.). (1992). Otoacoustic emissions. *Seminars in Hearing, 13*(1), 1–104.

DeConde Johnson, C. (1992). Section 504 of the Rehabilitation Act of 1973: Implications for audiology. *Educational Audiology Association Newsletter, 9*(2), 9–12.

Developmental approach to successful listening II (DASL II). (1989). Englewood, CO: Resource Point.

Dobie, R. A., & Berlin, C. I. (1979). Influence of otitis media on hearing and development. *Annals of Otology, Rhinology and Laryngology, 88*, 46–53.

Downs, M. P. (1980). Identification of children at risk for middle ear effusion problems. *Annals of Otology, Rhinology and Laryngology, 89*, 168–171.

Downs, M. P. (1988). Contribution of mild hearing loss to auditory language learning problems. In R. J. Roeser & M. P. Downs (Eds.), *Auditory disorders in school children* (2nd ed., pp. 186–199). New York: Thieme Medical Publishers.

Downs, M. P., Jafek, B., & Wood, R. P. (1981). Comprehensive treatment of children with recurrent serous otitis media. *Otolaryngology—Head and Neck Surgery, 89*, 658–665.

Draf, W., & Schulz, P. (1980). Insertion of ventilation tubes into the middle ear: Result and complications—A seven year review. *Annals of Otology, Rhinology and Laryngology, 89*, 303–307.

DuBow, S., Geer, S., & Strauss, K. P. (1992). *Legal rights: The guide for deaf and hard of hearing people* (4th ed.). Washington, DC: Gallaudet University Press.

Early intervention program for infants and toddlers with handicaps; final regulations. (1989). *Federal Register, 54*, (119), 26306–26348.

Education for all Handicapped Children Act of 1975, P.L. 94–142. (1975, November 29), *United States Statutes at Large, 89*, 773–796.

Education of Handicapped Children, P.L. 94–142 Regulations. (1977, August 23). *Federal Register, 42*(163), 42474–42518.

Education of the Handicapped Act Amendments of 1986, P.L. 99–457. (1986, October 8), *United States Statutes at Large, 100*, 1145–1177.

Education of the Handicapped Act Amendments of 1990, P.L. 101–476. (1990, October 30), *United States Statutes at Large, 104*, 1103–1151.

Edwards, C. (1991). Assessment and management of listening skills in school-aged children. In C. Flexer (Ed.), Current audiologic issues in the educational management of children with hearing loss, *Seminars in Hearing, 12*, 389–401.

Eichhorn, S. A. (1982). Congenital cytomegalovirus infection: A significant cause of deafness and mental deficiency. *American Annals of the Deaf, 127*, 838–842.

Eisenberg, R. B. (1976). *Auditory competence in early life*. Baltimore: University Park Press.

Elliott, L. L., Hammer, M. A., & Scholl, M. E. (1989). Fine grained auditory discrimination in normal children and children with language-learning problems. *Journal of Speech and Hearing Research, 32*, 112–119.

Erber, N. (1982). *Auditory training*. Washington, DC: The Alexander Graham Bell Association for the Deaf.

Ernst, M. (Ed.). (1997). Using audition to develop spoken language in children with severe and profound hearing loss. *Seminars in Hearing, 18*, 213–310.

Estabrooks, W. (Ed.). (1994). *Auditory-verbal therapy for parents and professionals*. Washington, DC: The Alexander Graham Bell Association for the Deaf.

Estabrooks, W. (Ed.). (1998). *Cochlear implants for kids*. Washington, DC: The Alexander Graham Bell Association for the Deaf.

Estabrooks, W., & Edwards, C. (1986). *Sure we can hear*. [Videotape]. Toronto, Canada: VOICE for Hearing-Impaired Children.

Estabrooks, W., & Schwartz, R. (1995). *The ABC's of AVT: Analyzing auditory-verbal therapy*. [Manual and videotape]. (Available from North York General Hospital, Learning to Listen Foundation, Toronto, Canada)

Evans, W., Webster, D., & Cullen, J. (1983). Auditory brainstem responses in neonatally sound deprived CBA/J mice. *Hearing Research, 10*, 269–277.

Feigin, J. A., & Stelmachowicz, P. G. (Eds.). (1991). *Pediatric amplification: Proceedings of the 1991 national conference*. Omaha, NE: Boys Town National Research Hospital.

Finitzo-Hieber, T., & Tillman, T. (1978). Room acoustics effects on monosyllabic word discrimination ability for normal and hearing-impaired children. *Journal of Speech and Hearing Research, 21*, 440–458.

Fisher, D. (1998). Elementary classrooms wired for listening/learning. *Educational Audiology Review, 15*, 4–5.

Flexer, C. (1989). Turn on sound: An odyssey of soundfield amplification. *Educational Audiology Association Newsletter, 5*, 6–7.

Flexer, C. (1991). Access to communication environments through assistive listening devices. *Journal of the Ohio Speech and Hearing Association, 6*, 9–14.

Flexer, C. (1992). FM classroom public address systems. In M. Ross (Ed.), *FM auditory training systems: Characteristics, selection, and use* (pp. 189–209). Parkton, MD: York Press.

Flexer, C. (1998). *Enhancing classrooms for listening, language and literacy.* [Videotape]. (Available from INFO-LINK Video Bulletin, Box 852, Layton, UT 84041, Telephone: [801] 544-1388)

Flexer, C., & Baumgarner, J. (1990). Guidelines for determining functional hearing in school-based settings. In M. J. Wilcox (Ed.), *Children with dual sensory impairment series*, Tallmadge, OH: Family Child Learning Center.

Flexer, C., & Gans, D. P. (1982). Evaluating behavioral observation audiometry with handicapped children. *Exceptional Child, 29*, 217–224.

Flexer, C., & Gans, D. P. (1983). Evaluating order of stimulus presentation with severe-profound multiply handicapped children using behavioral observation audiometry. *Ohio Journal of Speech and Hearing, 16*, 11–15.

Flexer, C., & Gans, D. P. (1985). Comparative evaluation of the auditory responsiveness of normal infants and profoundly multihandicapped children. *Journal of Speech and Hearing Research, 28*, 163–168.

Flexer, C., & Gans, D. P. (1986). Distribution of auditory response behaviors in normal infants and profoundly multihandicapped children. *Journal of Speech and Hearing Research, 29*, 425–429.

Flexer, C., & Ireland, J. (1986). Infant otitis media: A case study. *Hearing Instruments, 37*, 23–24, 50.

Flexer, C., Millin, J. P., & Brown, L. (1990). Children with developmental disabilities: The effect of soundfield amplification on word identification. *Language, Speech and Hearing Services in Schools, 21*, 177–182.

Flexer, C., Richards, C., Buie, C., & Brandy, W. (1994). Making the grade with amplification in classrooms. *Hearing Instruments, 45*, 24–26.

Flexer, C., & Savage, H. (1992). Using an ALD in speech-language assessment and training. *The Hearing Journal, 45*(4), 26–35.

Flexer, C., & Wood, L. A. (1984). The hearing aid: Facilitator or inhibitor of auditory interaction. *Volta Review, 86*, 354–361.

Flexer, C., Wray, D. & Ireland, J. (1989). Preferential seating is NOT enough: Issues in classroom management of hearing-impaired students. *Language, Speech and Hearing Services in Schools, 20*, 11–21.

Foster, S. M., Bracket, D., & Maxon, A. B. (1997, April). *Cochlear implant users listening in noise: Benefits of sound-field amplification.* Poster session presented at the annual meeting of the American Academy of Audiology, Ft. Lauderdale, Florida.

Franklin, B. (1989a). *Final report: The effect of tactile aids on communication skills of children with dual sensory impairments* (Grant No. G008630416). Washington, DC: Office of Special Education.

Friel-Patti, S., Finitzo, T., Formby, E., & Brown, K. C. (1987). A prospective study of early middle ear disease and speech-language development. *Texas Journal of Audiology and Speech Pathology, 13*, 39–43.

Fritsch, M. H., & Sommer, A. (1991). *Handbook of congenital and early onset hearing loss.* New York: Igaku-Shoin Medical Publishers.

Fulton, R. T., & Lloyd, L. L. (1975). *Auditory assessment of the difficult-to-test.* Baltimore: Williams & Wilkins.

Furth, H. (1964). Research with the deaf: Implications for language and cognition. *Psychological Bulletin, 62*(2), 145–162.

Gans, D. P. (1987). Improving behavior observation audiometry testing and scoring procedures. *Ear and Hearing, 8*, 92–100.

Gans, D. P., & Flexer, C. (1982). Observer bias in the hearing testing of profoundly involved multiply handicapped children. *Ear and Hearing, 3*, 309–313.

Garrard, K. R., & Clark, B. S. (1985). Otitis media: The role of speech-language pathologists. *Asha, 26*, 35–39.

Geers, A., & Moog, J. (1989). Factors predictive of the development of literacy in profoundly hearing-impaired adolescents. *The Volta Review, 91*, 69–86.

Gilbertson, M., & Bramlett, R. K. (1998). Phonological awareness screening to identify at-risk readers: Implications for practitioners. *Language, Speech and Hearing Services in Schools, 29*, 109–116.

Goldberg, D. M. (1987). Auditory assessment and management of school-aged hearing-impaired students. *Texas Journal of Audiology and Speech Pathology, 13*, 13–18.

Goldberg, D. M. (Ed.). (1993). Special focus section: Auditory-Verbal. *The Volta Review. 95*, 181–263.

Goldberg, D. M., & Flexer, C. (1993). Outcome survey of auditory-verbal graduates: Study of clinical efficacy. *Journal of the American Academy of Audiology, 4*, 189–200.

Goldberg, D. M., & Lebahn, C. (1990, July). *Performance of auditory-verbal children on the TAC.* Poster session presentation at the Biennial Convention of the Alexander Graham Bell Association for the Deaf, Washington, DC.

Goldstein, M. (1939). *The acoustic method.* St. Louis: Laryngoscope Press.

Gravel, J. S., Kurtzberg, D., Stapells, D. R., Vaughan, H. G., & Wallace, I. (1989). Case studies. *Seminars in Hearing, 10*, 272–290.

Gravel, J. S., McCarton, C. M., & Ruben, R. J. (1988). Otitis media and NICU graduates: A one-year prospective study. *Pediatrics, 82*, 44–49.

Gravel, J. D., & Wallace, I. F. (1992). Listening and language at 4 years of age: Effects of early otitis media. *Journal of Speech and Hearing Research, 35*, 588–595.

Gravel, J. S., Wallace, I. F., & Abraham, S. (1991, November). *Communication sequelae of otitis media.* Presentation at the American Speech-Language-Hearing Convention, Atlanta, GA.

Halpern, J., Hosford-Dunn, H., & Malachowski, N. (1987). Four factors that accurately predict hearing loss in "high risk" neonates. *Ear and Hearing, 8*, 21–25.

Harada, T., & Sando, I. (1981). Temporal bone histopathologic findings in Down's Syndrome. *Archives of Otolaryngology, 107*, 96–103.

Harrison, C. J., & Belhorn, T. H. (1991). Antibiotic treatment failures in acute otitis media. *Pediatric Annals, 20*, 600–608.

Hasselberger, W. (1998). MicroLink FM system: A review. *Educational Audiology Review, 15*, 20.

Hawkins, D. B. (1984). Comparisons of speech recognition in noise by mildly-to-moderately hearing-impaired children using hearing aids and FM systems. *Journal of Speech and Hearing Disorders, 49*, 409–418.

Hayes, D., & Northern, J. L. (1996). *Infants and hearing.* San Diego, CA: Singular Publishing Group.

Hood, L. J. (1998). *Clinical applications of the auditory brainstem response.* San Diego, CA: Singular Publishing Group.

Houtgast, T., & Steeneken, H. J. M. (1985). The MTF concept in room acoustics and its use for estimating speech intelligibility in auditoria. *Journal of Acoustical Society of America, 77*, 1069–1077.

Ingrao, B. (1997). Stick it in your ear: Earmolds revisited. *Educational Audiology Association Newsletter, 14*, 20–22.

Jacobson, J. T. (1997). A review of genetic hearing loss. *The Hearing Journal, 50*, 10–21.

Jerger, J. (Ed.). (1984). *Pediatric audiology.* San Diego, CA: College-Hill Press.

Johnson , C. D., Benson , P. V., & Seaton, J. B. (1997). *Educational audiology handbook.* San Diego, CA: Singular Publishing Group.

Johnson, D. (1975). Communication characteristics of NTID students. *Journal of the Academy of Rehabilitative Audiology, 8*, 17–32.

Johnson, D. (1976). Communication characteristics of a young deaf adult population: Techniques for evaluating their communication skills. *American Annals of the Deaf, 121*(4), 409–424.

Johnson, J., & Newport, E. (1989). Critical period effects in second-language learning: The influence of maturational state on the acquisition of English as a second language. *Cognitive Psychology, 21*, 60–90.

Johnson, K. C., Williamson, W. D., & Chmiel, R. (1991). Management of hearing disorder resulting from cytomegalovirus. *Hearing Instruments, 42*, 20–22.

Johnson, W. W. (1961). A survey of middle ears: 101 autopsies of infants. *Annals of Otology, Rhinology and Laryngology, 70*, 377–402.

Kaga, K., & Marsh, R. R. (1986). Auditory brainstem responses in young children with Down's syndrome. *International Journal of Pediatric Otorhinolaryngology, 11*, 29–38.

Katoff, L., Reuter, J., & Dunn, V. (1978). *The Kent infant developmental scale manual.* Kent, OH: Kent State University.

Kinney, J. S., Onorato, I. M., & Stewart J. A. (1985). Cytomegaloviral infection and disease. *Journal of Infectious Diseases, 151*, 772–774.

Kraus, N., Ozdamar, O., Heydemann, P. T., Stein, L., & Reed, N. (1984). Auditory brainstem responses in hydrocephalic patients. *Electroencephalography and Clinical Neurophysiology, 59,* 310–317.

Kretschmer, R. R., & Kretschmer, L. (1978). *Language development and intervention with the hearing impaired.* Baltimore: University Park Press.

Lasky E. (1983). Parameters affecting auditory processing. In E. Lasky & J. Katz (Eds.), *Central auditory processing disorders: Problems of speech, language, learning* (pp. 11–29). Baltimore: University Park Press.

Lass, N., Carlin, M., Woodford, C., Campanelli-Humphreys, A., Judy, S., Hushion-Stemple, E., & Boggs, J. (1986). A survey of professionals' knowledge of and exposure to hearing loss. *Volta Review, 88,* 333–338.

Leavitt, R. J. (1987). Promoting the use of rehabilitation technology. *Asha, 29,* 28–31.

Leavitt, R. J. (1991). Group amplification systems for students with hearing impairment. In C. Flexer (Ed.), Current audiologic issues in the educational management of children with hearing loss, *Seminars in Hearing, 12,* 380–388.

Leavitt, R. J. (1996). A consumer's guide to hearing aids. In C. Flexer, D. Wray, R. Leavitt, & R. Flexer, (Eds.), *How the student with hearing loss can succeed in college: A handbook for students, families, and professionals* (2nd ed., pp. 61–84). Washington, DC: The Alexander Graham Bell Association for the Deaf.

Leavitt, R. J., & Flexer, C. (1991). Speech degradation as measured by the rapid speech transmission index (RASTI). *Ear and Hearing, 12,* 115–118.

Lennenberg, E. (1967). *Biologic foundations of language.* New York: John Wiley.

Leonard, L. B. (1991, April). New trends in the study of early language acquisition. *Asha, 33,* 43–44.

Liden, G., & Kankkunen, A. (1969). Visual reinforcement audiometry. *Acta Otolaryngologica, 67,* 281–292.

Ling, D. (1976). *Speech and the hearing impaired child: Theory and Practice.* Washington, DC: The Alexander Graham Bell Association for the Deaf.

Ling, D. (1986). On auditory learning. *Newsounds, 11,* 1.

Ling, D. (1989). *Foundations of spoken language for hearing impaired children.* Washington, DC: The Alexander Graham Bell Association for the Deaf.

Ling, D. (1997). *Acoustics, audition and speech reception.* [Videotape]. (Available from Auditory-Verbal International, Inc. (AVI), 2121 Eisenhower Avenue, Suite 402. Alexandria, VA 22314. Telephone: [703] 739-1049)

Ling, D., & Ling, A. (1978). *Aural habilitation: The foundations of verbal learning in hearing-impaired children.* Washington, DC: The Alexander Graham Bell Association for the Deaf.

Longbury-Martin, B. L., Whitehead, M. L., & Martin, G. K. (1991). Clinical applications of otoacoustic emissions. *Journal of Speech and Hearing Research, 34,* 964–981.

Lovas, D. S. (1986). Pre-school sound field amplification. *The Directive Teacher, 8*, 22–23.

Lowell, E., Rushford, G., Hoversten, G., & Stoner, M. (1956). Evaluation of pure-tone audiometry with pre-school age children. *Journal of Speech and Hearing Disorders, 21*, 292–302.

Luckner, J. L. (1991). Mainstreaming hearing-impaired students: Perceptions of regular educators. *Language, Speech and Hearing Services in Schools, 22*, 302–307.

Luetke-Stahlman, B., & Moeller, M. P. (1987, June). *Are parents trained to sign proficiently to their deaf children?* Presentation at the Academy of Rehabilitative Audiology Summer Institute, Uniontown, PA.

Lundeen, C. (1991). Prevalence of hearing impairment among school children. *Language, Speech and Hearing Services in Schools, 22*, 269–271.

MacDonald, J., & Gillette, Y. (1989). *Beginning partners with children: From play to conversation*. Chicago: Riverside Publishing.

Madell, J. (1990). Managing classroom amplification. In M. Ross (Ed.), *Hearing-impaired children in the mainstream*. Parkton, MD: York Press.

Madell, J. R., & Sandrock, C. (1997, June). Selecting an FM system: When a hearing instrument is not enough. *The Hearing Review*, pp. 8, 12, 16.

Manning, A. (1998, June 29). Women outpacing men by degrees. *USA Today*, p. 1.

Manning, A., Flexer, C., & Shackelford, L. (1991). The role of hearing in early language intervention for toddlers with Down syndrome: Input precedes output. *Journal of the Ohio Speech and Hearing Association, 6*, 51–53.

Marler, P. R. (1970). A comparative approach to vocal learning: Song development in white-crowned sparrows. *Journal of Comparative and Physiological Psychology Monographs, 71*(2, Part 2), 1–25.

Martin, F. N., Bernstein, M. E., Daly, J. A., & Cody, J. P. (1988). Classroom teachers' knowledge of hearing disorders and attitudes about mainstreaming hard-of-hearing children. *Language, Speech and Hearing Services in Schools, 19*, 83–95.

Martin, F. N. & Clark, J. G. (1996). *Hearing care for children*. Boston: Allyn and Bacon.

Matkin, N. (1981). Amplification for children: Current status and future priorities. In F. Bess, B. Freeman, & J. Sinclair (Eds.), *Amplification in education* (pp. 192–201). Washington, DC: Alexander Graham Bell Association for the Deaf.

Matkin, N. (1990, June). *Recognizing cultural diversity when counseling families of children with hearing impairment*. Presentation at Pediatric Audiology Update conference. Providence, RI.

Maurizi, M., Ottaviani, F., Paludetti, G., & Lungarotti, S. (1985). Audiological findings in Down's children. *International Journal of Pediatric Otorhinolaryngology, 9*, 227–232.

Maxon, A. B., & Smaldino, J. (1991). Hearing aid management for children. In C. Flexer (Ed.), Current audiologic issues in the educational management of children with hearing loss, *Seminars in Hearing, 12*, 365–379.

McCormick, B. (1993). *Pediatric audiology, 0–5 years* (2nd ed.). San Diego, CA: Singular Publishing Group.

McGee, D. (1990). Recognizing heterogeneity: Increasing educational opportunities through mainstreaming. In M. Ross (Ed.), *Hearing-impaired children in the mainstream* (pp. 197–211). Parkton, MD: York Press.

McLellan, M. S., & Webb, C. H. (1961). Ear studies in the newborn infant. *Journal of Pediatrics, 58*, 672–677.

Menyuk, P. (1977). Effects of hearing loss on language acquisition in the babbling stage. In B. F. Jaffe (Ed). *Hearing loss in children* (pp. 621–629). Baltimore: University Park Press.

Merzenich, M. M., & Kaas, J. H. (1982). Organization of mammalian somatosensory cortex following peripheral nerve injury. *Trends in Neuroscience, 5*, 434–436.

Miller, J. F. (1988). Facilitating speech and language development. In C. Tingey (Ed.), *Down syndrome* (pp. 119–133). Boston: College-Hill Press.

Miyamoto, R. T., Osberger, M. J., & Robbins, A. M. (1992). Longitudinal evaluation of communication skills of children with single- or multi-channel cochlear implants. *American Journal of Otology, 13*, 215–222.

Moodie, K. S., Seewald, R. C., & Sinclair, D. T. (1994). Procedure for predicting real-ear hearing aid performance in young children. *American Journal of Audiology, 3*, 23–31.

Moores, D. (1987). *Educating the deaf: Psychology, principles, and practices* (3rd ed.). Boston: Houghton Mifflin.

Moses, K. (1985). Dynamic intervention with families. In E. Cherow (Ed.), *Hearing-impaired children and youth with developmental disabilities: An interdisciplinary foundation for service* (pp. 82–98). Washington, DC: Gallaudet College Press.

Mueller, H. G., & Killion, M. C. (1990). An easy method for calculating the articulation index. *The Hearing Journal, 43*, 14–22.

Musiek, F. E., & Berge, B. E. (1998). A neuroscience view of auditory training/stimulation and central auditory processing disorders. In M. G. Masters, N. A. Stecker, & J. Katz (Eds.), *Central auditory processing disorders: Mostly management* (pp. 15–32). Boston: Allyn and Bacon.

Myer, C. M., Farrer, S. M., Drake, A. F., & Cotton, R. T. (1989). Perilymphatic fistulas in children: Rationale for therapy. *Ear and Hearing, 10*, 112–116.

Myklebust, H. (1954). *Auditory disorders in children*. New York: Grune & Stratton.

Myklebust, H., & Brutton, M. (1953). A study of visual perception in deaf children. *Acta Oto-Laryngologica*, Suppl. 105, 1–126.

Neuss, D., Blair, J., & Viehweg, S. (1991). Sound field amplification: Does it improve word recognition in a background of noise for students with minimal hearing impairments? *Educational Audiology Monograph, 2*, 43–52.

Nevitt, A., & Brelsford, J. (1987). Effective audiological management of hearing-impaired children. *Texas Journal of Audiology and Speech Pathology, 13*, 5–13.

Newport, E. (1990). Maturational constraints on language learning. *Cognitive Science, 14*, 11–28.

Niskar, A. S., Kieszak, S. M., Holmes, A., Esteban, E., Rubin, C., & Brody, D. J. (1998). Prevalence of hearing loss among children 6 to 19 years: The third National Health and Nutrition Examination Survey. *Journal of the American Medical Association (JAMA), 279*, 1071–1075.

Northern, J. L. (Ed.). (1996). *Hearing disorders* (3rd ed.). Needham Heights, MA: Allyn & Bacon.

Northern, J. L., & Downs, M. P. (1991). *Hearing in children* (4th ed.). Baltimore: Williams & Wilkins.

Nozza, R. J., Rossman, R. N. F., Bond, L. C., & Miller, S. L. (1990). Infant speech-sound discrimination in noise. *Journal of the Acoustical Society of America, 87*, 339–350.

Olsen, W. O., Hawkins, D. B., & VanTassell, D. J. (1987). Representatives of the longterm spectrum of speech. *Ear and Hearing, 8*(5, Suppl.), 100–108.

Osberger, M. J. (1990, April). Audiological rehabilitation with cochlear implants and tactile aids. *Asha, 32*(4), 38–43.

Osberger, M. J., Maso, M., & Sam, L. K. (1993). Speech intelligibility of children with cochlear implants, tactile aids, or hearing aids. *Journal of Speech and Hearing Research, 36*, 186–203.

Osborn, J., Graves, L., & VonderEmbse, D. (1989). [Three-year sound field study in Putnam County, Ohio]. Unpublished raw data.

Oyler, R. F., Oyler, A. L., & Matkin, N. D. (1988). Unilateral hearing loss: Demographics and educational impact. *Language, Speech and Hearing Services in Schools, 19*, 201–210.

Paden, E. P., Novak, M. A., & Beiter, A. L. (1987). Predictors of phonologic inadequacy in young children prone to otitis media. *Journal of Speech and Hearing Disorders, 52*, 232–242.

Palmer, C. (1996, April). *Quantification of the ecobehavioral impact of a soundfield system.* Poster session presented at the annual meeting of the American Academy of Audiology, Salt Lake City, Utah.

Palmer, C. V. (1997). Hearing and listening in a typical classroom. *Language, Speech and Hearing Services in Schools, 28*, 213–218.

Pappas, D. G. (1998). *Diagnosis and treatment of hearing impairment in children* (2nd ed.). San Diego, CA: Singular Publishing Group.

Pappas, D. G., Flexer, C., & Shackelford, L. (1994). Otological and habilitative management of children with Down syndrome. *Laryngoscope, 104*, 1065–1070.

Pappas, D. G., & Schneiderman, T. S. (1989). Perilymphatic fistula in pediatric patients with a preexisting sensorineural loss. *The American Journal of Otology, 10*, 499–501.

Paradise, J. L. (1980). Otitis media in infants and children (Review article). *Pediatrics, 65*, 917–943.

Paradise, J. L. (1981). Otitis media during early life: How hazardous to development? A critical review of the evidence (Special article). *Pediatrics, 68*, 869–873.

Paradise, J. L., & Bluestone, C. D. (1974). Early treatment of the universal otitis media of children cleft palate. *Pediatrics, 53*, 48–54.

Paradise, J. L., Smith, C., & Bluestone, C. D. (1976). Tympanometric detection of middle ear effusion in infants and young children. *Pediatrics, 58*, 198–206.

Parents and Families of Natural Communication, Inc. (1998). *We CAN hear and speak! The power of auditory-verbal communication for children who are deaf or hard of hearing*. Washington, DC: The Alexander Graham Bell Association for the Deaf.

Parving, A. (1993). Congenital hearing disability: Epidemiology and identification: A comparison between two health authority districts. *International Journal of Pediatric Otolaryngology, 27*, 29–46.

Pashley, N. R. T. (1984). Otitis media. In J. L. Northern (Ed.), *Hearing disorders* (2nd ed., pp. 103–110). Boston: Little, Brown.

Patchett, T. A. (1977). Auditory discrimination in albino rats as a function of auditory restriction at different ages. *Developmental Psychology, 13*, 168–169.

Pediatric Working Group of the Conference on Amplification for Children with Auditory Deficits. (1996). Amplification for infants and children with hearing loss. *American Journal of Audiology, 5*, 53–68.

Pillai, P. (1997). Understanding the needs of hard of hearing students in a mainstream setting. *Perspectives in Education and Deafness, 15*, 10–11.

Pillow, G. (1998). New personal soundfield from Audio Enhancement: A review. *Educational Audiology Review, 15*, 20.

Pollack, D. (1970). *Educational audiology for the limited hearing infant*. Springfield, IL: Charles C Thomas.

Pollack, D. (1985). *Educational audiology for the limited hearing infant and preschooler* (2nd ed.). Springfield, IL: Charles C Thomas.

Pollack, D., Goldberg, D., & Caleffe-Schenck, N. (1997). *Educational audiology for the limited-hearing infant and preschooler: An auditory-verbal program* (3rd ed.). Springfield, IL: Charles C Thomas.

Primus, M. A. (1987). Response and reinforcement in operant audiometry. *Journal of Speech and Hearing Disorders, 52*, 294–299.

Ray, H., Sarff, L. S., & Glassford, F. E. (1984). Soundfield amplification: An innovative educational intervention for mainstreamed learning disabled students. *The Directive Teacher, 6*, 18–20.

Rehabilitation Act Amendments of 1992, P.L. 102–569. (1992, October 29). *United States Statutes at Large, 106*, 4344–4488.

Rehabilitation Act of 1973, P.L. 93–112. (1973, September 26). *United States Statutes at Large, 87*, 355–394.

Rehabilitation, Comprehensive Services, and Developmental Disabilities Amendments of 1978. (P.L. 95-602. November 6, 1978). *United States Statutes at Large, 92*, 2955–3017.

Reichman, J., & Healey, W. C. (1983). Learning disabilities and conductive hearing loss involving otitis media. *Journal of Learning Disabilities, 16*, 272–278.

Robertson, D., & Irvine, D. R. F. (1989). Plasticity of frequency organization in auditory cortex of guinea pigs with partial unilateral deafness. *Journal of Comparative Neurology, 282*, 456–471.

Robertson L., & Flexer, C. (1993). Reading development: A parent survey of children with hearing impairment who developed speech and language through the auditory-verbal method. *The Volta Review, 95*(3), 253–261.

Roeser, R. J., & Crandell, C. (1991). The audiologist's responsibility in cerumen management. *Asha, 33*(1), 51–53.

Ross, M. (Ed.). (1990). *Hearing-impaired children in the mainstream.* Parkton, MD: York Press.

Ross, M. (1991). A future challenge: Educating the educators and public about hearing loss. In C. Flexer (Ed.), Current audiologic issues in the educational management of children with hearing loss, *Seminars in Hearing, 12*, 402–413.

Ross, M. (Ed.). (1992). *FM auditory training systems: Characteristics, selection and use.* Timonium, MD: York Press.

Ross, M., Brackett, D., & Maxon, A. (1982). *Hard of hearing children in regular schools.* Englewood Cliffs, NJ: Prentice-Hall.

Ross, M., Brackett, D., & Maxon, A. (1991). *Assessment and management of mainstreamed hearing-impaired children.* Austin, TX: Pro-Ed.

Ross, M., & Calvert, D. R. (1984). Semantics of deafness revisited: Total communication and the use and misuse of residual hearing. *Audiology, 9*, 127–145.

Ross, M., & Giolas, T. G. (Eds.). (1978). *Auditory management of hearing-impaired children.* Baltimore: University Park Press.

Ross, M., & Leavitt, H. (1998). Telecoils ("T" coils) and direct audio input (DAI). *Volta Voices, 5*, 10.

Rowe, L. D. (1985, October). Hearing loss: The profound benefits of early diagnosis. *Contemporary Pediatrics, 2*, 78–85.

Ruben, R. J., & Math, R. (1978). Serous otitis media associated with sensorineural hearing loss in children. *Laryngoscope, 88*, 1139–1154.

Savage, H., & Flexer, C. (1987, March). *Communication—Are you listening?* Presentation at a National Interdisciplinary Seminar on Down syndrome, sponsored by Blick Clinic for Developmental Disabilities, Akron, OH.

Seaton, J., & Lewis, D. (1997). BTE-FM: The future is now! *Educational Audiology Association Newsletter, 14*, 3–6.

Seewald, R. C. (1992). The desired sensation level method for fitting children: Version 3.0. *Hearing Journal, 45*, 36–41.

Sehgal, S. T., Kirk, K. I., Svirsky, M., Ertmer, D. J., & Osberger, M. J. (1998). Imitative consonant feature production by children with multichannel sensory aids. *Ear and Hearing, 19*, 72–84.

Sehgal, S.T., Kirk, K.I., Svirsky, M., & Miyamoto, R.T. (1998). The effects of processor strategy on the speech perception performance of pediatric nucleus multichannel cochlear implant users. *Ear and Hearing, 19,* 149–161.

Self Help for Hard of Hearing People. (1992). *Getting through "A guide to better understanding . . ."* [Audio tape]. Bethesda, MD: Author.

Sharpe, R. (1994, April 12). The early brain. *Wall Street Journal.*

Sheehy, J. L. (1983). Dead ear? Not necessarily—A report of three cases of chronic otitis media. *American Journal of Otology, 4,* 238–239.

Silva, P. A., Chalmers, D., & Stewart, I. (1986). Some audiological, psychological, educational, and behavioral characteristics of children with bilateral otitis media with effusion: A longitudinal study. *Journal of Learning Disabilities, 19,* 165–169.

Simon, C. S. (1985). *Communication skills and classroom success.* San Diego, CA: College-Hill Press.

Sindrey, D. (1997). *Listening games for littles.* London, Ontario, Canada: Word Play Publications.

Snow, J. B. (1979). Otoneurologic evaluation. In W. F. Rintelmann (Ed.), *Hearing assessment* (pp. 101–131). Baltimore: University Park Press.

Sprague, B. H., Wiley, T. L., & Goldstein, R. (1985). Tympanometric and acoustic-reflex studies in neonates. *Journal of Speech and Hearing Research, 28,* 265–272.

Stach, B. A. (1998). *Clinical audiology: An introduction.* San Diego, CA: Singular Publishing Group.

Stein, D. M. (1983). Psychosocial characteristics of school-age children with unilateral hearing loss. *Journal of the Academy of Rehabilitative Audiology, 16,* 12–22.

Strome, M. (1981). Down's syndrome: A modern otorhinolaryngological perspective. *Laryngoscope. 91,* 1581–1594.

Studebaker, G. A., Bess, F. H., & Beck, L. B. (Eds.). (1991). *The Vanderbilt hearing aid report II.* Baltimore, MD: York Press.

Sudler, W. H., & Flexer, C. (1986). Low cost assistive listening device. *Language, Speech and Hearing Services in Schools, 17,* 342–344.

Suzuki, T., & Ogiba, Y. (1961). Conditioned orientation audiometry. *Archives of Otolaryngology, 74,* 192–198.

Swigonski, N., Shallop, J., Bull, M. J., & Lemons, J. A. (1987). Hearing screening of high risk newborns. *Ear and Hearing, 8,* 26–30.

Teele, D. W. (1991). Strategies to control recurrent acute otitis media in infants and children. *Pediatric Annals, 20,* 609–616.

Tos, M., Holm-Jensen, S., Sorensen, C. H., & Morgensen, C. (1982). Spontaneous course and frequency of secretory otitis in 4-year-old children. *Archives of Otolaryngology, 108,* 4–11.

Trelease, J. (1995). *The read aloud handbook.* Fairfield, PA: Penguin Books.

Tucker, B. P. (1998a). *Cochlear implants: A handbook.* McFarland & Company, Inc.

Tucker, B. P. (1998b). *IDEA advocacy for children who are deaf or hard of hearing.* San Diego: Singular Publishing Group.

Tye-Murray, N. (1998). Foundations of aural rehabilitation. San Diego, CA: Singular Publishing Group.

Tyler, R. T. (1993). *Cochlear implants*. San Diego: Singular Publishing Group.

Tyler, R. S., Moore, B., & Kuk, F. (1989). Performance of some of the better cochlear-implant patients. *Journal of Speech and Hearing Research, 32*, 887–911.

United States Department of Health and Human Services. (1994). *Clinical practice guidelines: Otitis media with effusion in young children.* (AHCPR NO. 94–0622; Telephone: [800] 358-9295)

Upfold, L. J. (1988). Children with hearing aids in the 1980's: Etiologies and severity of impairment. *Ear and Hearing, 9*, 75–80.

Urbantschitsch, V. (1982). *Auditory training for deaf mutism and acquired deafness* (S. R. Silverman, trans.). Washington, DC: The Alexander Graham Bell Association for the Deaf.

Valente, M. (1998). The bright promise of microphone technology. *The Hearing Journal, 51*, 10–19.

VanTasell, D. J., Mallinger, C. A., & Crump, E. S. (1986). Functional gain and speech recognition with two types of F.M. amplification. *Language, Speech and Hearing Services in Schools, 17*, 28–37.

Vaughan, P. (1981). *Learning to listen*. New York: Bequfort Books.

Vaughn, G. R., Lightfoot, R. K., & Gibbs, S. D. (1983). Assistive listening devices. Part III: Space. *Asha, 25*, 33–46.

Ventry, I. M. (1980). Effects of conductive hearing loss: Fact or fiction. *Journal of Speech and Hearing Disorders, 45*, 143-156.

Warren, W. S., & Stool, S. E. (1971). Otitis media in low birth-weight infants. *Journal of Pediatrics, 79*, 740–743.

Webster, D. (1983). A critical period during postnatal auditory development of mice. *International Journal of Pediatric Otorhinolaryngology, 6*, 107–118.

Weisenberger, J. M., & Miller, J. D. (1987). The role of tactile aids in providing information about acoustic stimuli. *Journal of the Acoustical Society of America, 82*, 906–916.

White, K. R., & Behrens, T. R. (Eds.). (1993). The Rhode Island hearing assessment project: Implications for universal newborn hearing screening. *Seminars in Hearing, 14*(1), 1–122.

White, T. P., Hoffman, S. R., & Gale, E. N. (1986). Psychophysiological therapy for tinnitus. *Ear and Hearing, 7*, 397–399.

Williamson, W. D., Percy, A. K., Yow, M. D., Gerson, P., Catlin, F. I., Koppelman, M. L., & Thurber, S. (1990). Asymptomatic congenital cytomegalovirus infection: Audiologic, neuroradiologic and neurodevelopmental abnormalities during the first year. *American Journal of Disabled Child, 144*, 1365–1368.

Wray, D., Hazlett, J., & Flexer, C. (1988). Strategies for teaching writing skills to hearing-impaired adolescents. *Language, Speech and Hearing Services in Schools, 19*, 182–190.

Wright, C. G. (1997). Development of the human external ear. *Journal of the American Academy of Audiology, 8,* 379–382.

Yoshinaga-Itano, C., & Pollack, D. (1988). *A description of children in the acoupedic method and a retrospective study of the acoupedic method.* Denver, CO: The Listen Foundation.

Zabel, H., & Tabor, M. (1993). Effects of classroom amplification on spelling performance of elementary school children. *Educational Audiology Monograph, 3,* 5–9.

Zimmerman-Phillips, S., Osberger, M. J., & Robbins, A. M. (1997). *Infant-toddler meaningful auditory integration scale (IT-MAIS).* Sylmer, CA: Advanced Bionics Corporation.

Glossary of Terms Used by Audiologists

Accommodations: Services or equipment to which the student with a disability legally is entitled for the purpose of providing an adequate and equitable education.

Acoustic: Sound, its physical nature.

Acoustic filter effect of hearing impairment: Hearing impairment acts like an invisible acoustic filter that distorts, smears, or eliminates incoming sounds; the negative impact of this filter on spoken communication, reading, academics, and independent function causes the problems associated with hearing impairment.

Acoustic phonetics: The study of speech sounds as they are perceived by the ear of the listener; objective study and measurement of the sound waves produced when speech sounds are spoken.

Acoustical treatment: Using a material or process for changing the absorptive or reflective characteristics of a surface in a room.

Acoustically modified earmolds: Specifically shaped earmolds that change the output of the hearing aid (e.g., Libby Horn shape which improves high-frequency amplification).

Acquired hearing impairment: Hearing impairments that occur after speech and language have been developed.

Aided thresholds: Represented by the symbol "A" on an audiogram, they are the softest tones that a person can hear while wearing hearing aids.

Air conduction: Sound travels through the air from a source, reaches the ear, enters the auditory system through the ear canal, and progresses through the eardrum, middle ear, inner ear, and then to the brain. Air conduction thresholds are obtained by using the earphones of an audiometer, with the symbol "O" representing right ear sensitivity and the symbol "X" representing left ear sensitivity on an audiogram.

Ambient noise: Sounds in the environment that are not a part of the desired acoustic signal.

Amplifier: A device that increases the intensity of an electrical signal.

Amplification: To make sounds louder; may also refer to a piece of equipment used to make sounds louder, such as a hearing aid.

Assistive listening device (ALD): Any of a number of pieces of equipment used to augment hearing or to assist the hearing aid in difficult listening situations; through the use of a remote microphone, assistive listening devices provide a superior signal-to-noise ratio that enhances the clarity (intelligibility) of the speech signal.

Atresia: Absence or complete closure of the ear canal, causing a conductive-type hearing impairment.

Attention span: The length of time that a person can concentrate on a task without distraction.

Attenuation: A reduction or decrease in magnitude; a sound made softer.

Audibility: Being able to hear but not necessarily distinguish among speech sounds.

Audiogram: A graph of a person's peripheral hearing sensitivity with frequency (pitch) on one axis and intensity (loudness) on the other.

Audiologist: An individual who holds a graduate degree, state license, and professional certification for the assessment and management of hearing and hearing problems.

Audiometer: An instrument that delivers calibrated pure tone or speech stimuli for the measurement of sound detection and speech detection, recognition, and identification.

Auditory background: An unconscious (primitive) function of hearing that allows identification of sounds that are consistent with specific locations (e.g., schools, grocery stores, hospitals) and biological functions.

Auditory behaviors: Behaviors displayed by infants and children in response to acoustic stimulation; may be categorized as being attentive or reflexive in nature.

Auditory brainstem response (ABR): An objective test that measures the tiny electrical potentials produced in response to sound stimuli by the synchronous discharge of the first- through sixth-order neurons in the auditory nerve and brain stem.

Auditory system: A term used to describe the entire structure and function of the ear.

Autoimmune: This term refers to a disordered immunologic response in which the body produces antibodies against its own tissues; may occur in the inner ear.

Background noise: Any unwanted sound that may or may not interfere with listening depending on the speech-to-noise ratio in the environment.

Behavioral observation audiometry (BOA): The "lowest" developmental level test procedure whereby a controlled, calibrated sound stimulus is presented, and an infant's or child's *unconditioned* response behaviors are observed.

Behavioral tests: Hearing tests that elicit a behavior, measure that behavior, and infer function of the auditory system.

Bilateral: A disorder or hearing loss that involves both ears.

Binaural: Hearing with both ears; wearing a separate hearing aid on each ear.

Bone conduction: A pathway by which sounds directly reach the inner ear primarily through skull vibration, thereby bypassing the outer and middle ears.

Bone oscillator: The piece of audiometric equipment that looks like a small black box attached to a headband and is used to obtain bone conduction thresholds.

Button receiver: A small circular sound transducer that is attached to a snap-ring earmold.

Calibrate: To check or adjust a piece of equipment until it accurately conforms to a predetermined, standard measure.

Central auditory processing disorder (CAPD): Not really a hearing impairment relative to impairment of reception, central auditory problems cause difficulty with perception or deriving meaning from incoming sounds. The source of the problem is in the central auditory nervous system (brain stem or cortex) not in the peripheral hearing mechanism (outer, middle, or inner ear).

Central mechanism: The part of the ear structure that includes the brain stem and cortex.

Certified Auditory-Verbal Therapist (Cert. AVT): Audiologists, speech-language pathologists, or teachers of children with hearing impairments who have obtained additional supervised training beyond their typical degrees and who have passed a special certification examination for auditory-verbal therapists; a registry of Cert. AVTs may be obtained from Auditory-Verbal International, Inc. (AVI).

Cerumen: Also called ear wax. A normal, protective secretion of the ear canal. Approximately 30% of infants and young children in early intervention programs have so much ear wax that it causes a hearing impairment that interferes with the learning of language (spoken communication).

Classroom acoustics: The noise and reverberation (echo) characteristics of a classroom as determined by sound sources inside and outside the classroom, including classroom size, shape, surface material, furniture, persons, and other physical characteristics.

Clear speech: Speech that is spoken at a moderately loud conversational level, characterized by precise but not exaggerated articulation, pausing at appropriate places, and speaking at a somewhat slower rate; is easier for people with hearing loss to understand.

Cochlea: The inner ear where the reception of sound actually occurs. The organ of Corti (end-organ for hearing) and hair cells (sensory receptors for sound) are located in the cochlea.

Cochlear implant: A biomedical device that delivers electrical stimulation to the VIIIth cranial nerve (auditory nerve) via an electrode array surgically implanted in the cochlea.

Colloquial terms: Words or phrases used in everyday conversation that are typically learned by "overhearing."

Complex sound: A sound made up of two or more frequencies.

Compression (in hearing aid circuitry): Nonlinear amplifier gain used to determine the output of the signal from the hearing aid as a function of the input signal.

Conductive hearing impairment: Hearing impairment caused by damage or disease (pathology) located in the outer or middle ear that interferes with the efficient transmission of sound into the inner ear where sound reception occurs.

Conductive mechanism: The part of the auditory system that includes the outer and middle ear.

Congenital hearing impairment: A hearing impairment that occurs prior to the development of speech and language, usually before or at birth.

Consonant: A speech sound formed by restricting, channeling, or directing air flow with the tongue, teeth, and/or lips (e.g., th, s, p, f, m, and so on).

Coupled: The connecting or attaching of one object to another, for example, a hearing aid to an assistive listening device.

Decibel (db): The logarithmic unit of sound intensity or sound pressure; $\frac{1}{10}$th of a Bel.

Diagnostic audiologic assessment (hearing test): The collection of tests given to an individual who wants his or her hearing evaluated, typically including: case history, tuning forks, speech tests (threshold and word identification), pure tone air and bone conduction testing, impedance, and counseling.

Differential diagnosis: Separating peripheral hearing impairment from other problems that present with symptoms (e.g., lack of appropriate spoken language development and/or lack of appropriate and observable auditory behaviors) similar to hearing impairment.

Direct audio input (DAI): Direct transmission of a sound signal into a hearing aid without being changed from one form of energy to another.

Disability: Impairment or loss of function of whole or parts of body systems.

Discrimination: Ability to differentiate among sounds of different frequencies, durations, or intensities.

Distance hearing: The ability to monitor environmental events and to "overhear" conversations, an ability that is severely reduced by hearing impairment.

Distortion: Adding or taking away from the original form or composition of the acoustic signal.

Dynamic range compression circuits: Circuits in hearing aids designed to provide more amplification for soft sounds than for loud sounds to meet the needs of many hearing aid wearers, who primarily need more amplification of soft sounds.

Dysplasia (of the inner ear): Incomplete development or malformations of the inner ear (cochlea).

Ear canal: The canal between the pinna and eardrum, also called the external auditory meatus.

Earmold: The part of a hearing aid or ALD that fits into the ear and functions to conduct sound from the hearing aid into the ear.

Earshot: The distance over which (speech) sounds are intelligible; this distance is reduced when someone has a hearing loss.

Echo: A reflected sound that is perceived after the direct sound that initiated it.

Electroacoustic: Pertains to the electronic processing of sound.

Electrophysiologic tests: Tests that measure the electrical activity of the brain stem and brain in response to acoustic stimulation.

Endogenous hearing impairment: A hearing impairment caused by genetic factors that have various probabilities of being passed on to children or to grandchildren.

Environmental sounds: Nonspeech sounds such as a fire engine siren, a telephone ringing, the garage door opening, or a doorbell ringing.

Etiology: Cause of the hearing loss.

Exogenous hearing impairment: A hearing impairment caused by environmental factors such as a virus, medications, or lack of oxygen; cannot be passed on to offspring.

Feedback (acoustic): A high-pitched squeal produced by a hearing aid and caused most often by a poorly fitting earmold. Feedback also can be caused by cracked earmold tubing, earwax in the earmold, or a crack in the earhook or hearing-aid case.

Frequency: The number of times that any regularly repeated event, such as sound vibration, occurs in a specified period of time, usually measured in cycles per second. Also called pitch and measured in Hertz (Hz) along the top of an audiogram from low to high-frequency sounds; low-frequency sounds are most commonly associated with vowel sounds and high-frequency sounds with consonants.

Frequency modulation (FM): The frequency of transmitted waves is alternated in accordance with the sounds being sent; radio waves.

Frequency response: The way that each hearing aid or ALD shapes the incoming (speech) sounds to best reach the persons's hearing impairment; the amount of amplification provided by the hearing aid at any frequency.

Functional hearing impairment: A hearing problem with no physiological basis.

Gain: The amount by which the output level of the hearing aid or ALD exceeds the input level, how much louder sounds are made by an amplification device.

Hearing age (also called listening age): The relationship between the age of a child when he or she first receives amplification and that child's chronological age; for example a 3-year-old child is 1 day old relative to listening, language, and information learning when his or her hearing aids are first fit.

Hearing aids: Miniature public address systems that amplify and shape incoming sounds to make them audible to an ear that would not otherwise detect them; the first step in an aural habilitative procedure.

Hearing aid adjustment: Varying the controls of a hearing aid or the acoustics of an earmold to improve their capability to assist a specific person with a particular hearing impairment.

Hearing aid fitting: Trying a hearing aid and earmold on a person, using specific procedures, until it is suitable for the person acoustically, physically, and cosmetically.

Hearing aid programmability: Refers to a hearing aid's adjustment capability. If a hearing aid is *programmable*, its amplification characteristics can be fine-tuned to the hearing aid wearer's needs by use of a hand-held or personal computer interface. If the hearing-aid user's hearing changes, the hearing aid can be easily and quickly reprogrammed.

Hearing aid stethoscope: An instrument that allows one to listen to the output of a hearing aid or an ALD to detect a malfunction.

Hearing impairment: Lessened or loss of hearing sensitivity caused by disease or damage to one or more parts of one or both ears.

Hertz (Hz): A unit of frequency measurement equal to 1 cycle per second.

Horn, acoustic (of an earmold): Progressive increase of the internal diameter of the earmold sound channel resulting in a "horn effect" that enhances certain sounds. A common use is to restore some of the sound energy associated with ear canal resonance that may be lost when a conventional earmold is inserted into the ear.

IDEA—Individuals With Disabilities Education Act: Federal legislation to guarantee that all infants and children with disabilities receive a free, appropriate, public education that emphasizes special education and related services designed to meet their unique needs; the rights of children with disabilities and their parents or guardians are protected; and states are assisted in providing for the effective education of all children with disabilities. The most recent legislation is the IDEA Amendments of 1997.

Idioms: The assignment of a new meaning to a group of words that already have their own meaning, with the literal meaning no longer serving as the proper interpretation. For example, "a pain in the neck" does not mean that the person is physically ill but, rather, that the person is bothersome to another.

Idiopathic: No known cause (of the hearing loss).

IEP (Individualized Educational Plan): A legal, written contract developed by a team (school and parents) that specifies instructional and related services needed for the child to obtain an appropriate education; includes short- and long-term objectives.

IFSP (Individualized Family Service Plan): A written, legal document that describes a plan for services for infants, toddlers, and their families; the focus of this plan is the family rather than the individual child.

Impedance (immittance) testing: An objective measure of middle-ear function, not hearing sensitivity; measures how well the ear drum moves.

Inner ear: Comprised of the cochlea, which contains hair cells, the thousands of tiny receptors of sound, the vestibular or balance system, and the acoustic nerve that transmits nerve impulses from the inner ear to the brain.

Intelligibility: The ability to detect differences among speech sounds (e.g., to hear words such as "vacation" and "invitation" as separate and distinct words).

Intensity: Intensity also is referred to as loudness and is measured in dB.

Internal noise: Noise generated within a sound system such as a hearing aid or assistive listening device.

Intonation: Variations in pitch patterns (melody) and stress in an utterance that add meaning to the message.

Inverse square law: The intensity or loudness of a sound decreases 6 dB as the distance between the sound and the receiver is doubled.

Jack: An electrical device that can receive a plug to make a connection in a circuit (e.g., an amplifier that has a specific place where earphones can be attached to the unit).

Language: A structured symbolic system used to communicate ideas in the form of words, with rules for combining and sequencing these words into thoughts, experiences, or feelings. An oral language system is comprised of a sound system, a vocabulary or concept system, a word ordering and grammar system, and rules for effectively using this symbolic system.

Learning disability: The lack of a skill in one or more areas of learning that is inconsistent with the child's overall intellectual capacity.

Listening: Understanding speech and environmental sounds by attending to auditory clues; detection, discrimination, recognition, identification, and comprehension of speech and environmental sounds.

Listening age: *See* Hearing age.

Live signal: An unrecorded sound or voice.

Localization: The ability to determine where a sound is coming from; to associate a sound with a source by finding the source.

Loop FM system: A frequency modulated (FM) system that features magnetic (loop) induction and telecoil reception of the transmitted signal.

Loudness: The perception of sound intensity; marked by high volume.

Loudspeaker: An electroacoustic transducer that changes electrical energy into acoustical energy at the output stage of a sound system so that it can be heard by many persons at the same time.

Mainstreaming: The process that promotes integration in a general school setting and curriculum of the child with a disability to the maximum extent possible in accordance with Federal laws. Integration with typical children ranges from full-time placement to integration in classes like music, art, or gym.

Masking: A procedure often used in hearing testing where a static-like noise is presented to the nontest ear through headphones to keep it from responding to the test stimuli.

Maximum power output ([MPO]; also called Saturation sound pressure level [SSPL]): A hearing aid or ALD has a maximum output limit that cannot be exceeded regardless of how high the volume control is turned up or how loud the input sound becomes. If the SPL is set appropriately, it serves as a safety feature that prevents amplification devices from emitting uncomfortably loud or harmful sounds.

Microphone/transmitter: An electroacoustic transducer that changes a sound stimulus to electrical energy.

Middle ear: The part of the auditory mechanism that functions to conduct sound efficiently into the inner ear; made up of the eardrum, a small air-filled space, and the three smallest bones in the body.

Minimum response level (MRL): The lowest or softest in dB hearing level (dB HL) at which a baby displays identifiable behavioral changes to sound, usually considerably above or louder than his or her actual threshold.

Mixed hearing impairment: A hearing impairment caused by the presence of more than one pathology in different parts of the ear at the same time; it can be thought of as having two hearing impairments in the same ear, usually conductive and sensorineural.

Multifactoral inheritance: This means that there are additive effects of several minor gene-pair abnormalities in association with nongenetic environment interactive factors or "triggers," that cause hearing loss in a child.

Multiple-memory hearing aids: Offer different settings or memories for various listening environments. One memory may be used for quiet listening and another for listening in a noisy restaurant; a remote control is usually used to access the various memories. Ideally, each memory is adjusted to provide the hearing aid wearer with optimum hearing in that particular environment. Note that children MUST also have the remote microphone of an FM unit when in a classroom learning situation.

Neuropathy—auditory: A disorder of the auditory neural pathways including the VIIIth cranial (auditory) nerve, brain stem, and cortex.

Noise: Any unwanted or unintended sound or electrical signal that interferes with communication or transmission of energy; it may be disturbing and/or hazardous to hearing health.

Noise reduction: A process of acoustical treatments and structural modifications whereby the intensity in dB of unwanted sound is reduced in a room.

Objective tests: Objective tests provide some direct measurement of the auditory system (e.g., eardrum and middle ear mobility, middle ear muscle reflex action, and transmission of sound up the auditory pathways of the lower brainstem).

Occupied classroom: A classroom when the teacher and students are present.

Otitis media: Also known as middle ear infection, otitis media is the most common cause of conductive hearing impairment in children. It is an inflammation of the middle ear, typically with fluid present in the normally air-filled middle ear space.

Otoacoustic emissions (OAEs): Soft, inaudible sounds produced by vibratory motion of the (outer) hair cells in the cochlea. To measure evoked otoacoustic emissions, a small probe is inserted in the ear canal, sounds are presented, and response tracings are recorded.

Otologist: A physician who specializes in diseases of the ear; also known as an otolaryngologist or an Ear-Nose-Throat (ENT) specialist.

Ototoxicity: A "poisoning" of the delicate inner ear by high doses of certain drugs and medications.

Outer ear: The part of the hearing mechanism made up of the pinna and external auditory meatus (ear canal), that functions to protect and channel sounds into the middle ear.

Pediatric test battery: The use of several, developmentally appropriate behavioral and objective hearing tests with infants and children to avoid drawing conclusions from a single test, allow detection of multiple pathologies, and provide a framework for observation of auditory behaviors.

Perception: Understanding the meaning of incoming sounds; occurs in the central auditory system (brainstem and cortex).

Perilymphatic fistula: A leak in the oval or round windows, both being points of communication between the middle and inner ear; causes sudden or degenerative hearing impairments.

Peripheral auditory mechanism: The part of the ear that includes the outer, middle, and inner ear; it functions to receive incoming sounds.

Personal FM system: A radio system that delivers frequency modulated signals and has individual wearable receiver units.

Phonetic: Having to do with the phonemes or distinctive sounds that make up the words of a language.

Phonological awareness (phonemic awareness): The explicit awareness of the speech sound structure of language units that forms the basis for reading. It is demonstrated by a variety of skills that include generating rhyming words, segmenting words into syllables and into discrete sounds, and categorizing groups of words based on a similarity of sound segments.

Pinna: The auricle or outer flap of the ear; one located on each side of the head.

Play audiometry: The highest level of pediatric task in hearing testing, play audiometry involves the active cooperation of the child while an auditory stimulus is paired with an operant task, such as dropping a block in a bucket.

Pragmatics: The study of how language is used.

Prognosis: A prediction of the course or outcome of a disease or treatment.

Programmable hearing aid: *See* Hearing aid programmability.

Propagation: Act of extending, projecting, or traveling through space.

Prosodic: Stress, intonation, or melodic features of spoken language.

Pure tone: A tone that has energy at only one frequency. Pure tones are useful for evaluating hearing sensitivity because they permit measurement of the contour or configuration of the hearing impairment.

Rapid speech transmission index (RASTI): A number between zero and one that quantifies speech intelligibility. RASTI is derived from measurement of the modulation transfer function of two octave bands of pink noise modulations that mimic the long-term speech spectrum.

Real ear measurements: Measurement of amplified sound in the ear canal through the use of a probe microphone.

Reception: The detection of sound that occurs in the inner ear.

Receptive language: Skills involving the ability to receive and comprehend the language one hears in the environment.

Redundancy: The part of a message that can be eliminated without loss of information.

Reflected sound: Propagated sound after it has struck one or more objects or surfaces in a room.

Remote control: Hand-held device that permits adjustments in the volume or changes in the program of a programmable hearing aid.

Remote microphone: A microphone that can be placed close to the desired sound source, thereby improving the speech-to-noise ratio (S/N ratio); a key feature of FM systems, sound-field FM systems, and some hardwired assistive listening devices.

Residual hearing: The hearing that remains after damage or disease in the auditory mechanism; there is almost always some residual hearing, even with the most profound hearing impairments. Residual hearing can be accessed through the use of amplification technology.

Reverberant sound: Sound that reaches a given location in a room only after being reflected from one or more barriers or partitions within a room.

Reverberation: The amount of echo in a room; the more reverberant the room, the poorer the speech-to-noise ratio and the less intelligible the speech.

Secondary language: Skills that involve higher level language, such as reading and writing versus listening and speaking.

Segmental: Pertaining to the sounds of speech.

Semantic: Related to the meaning of words or groups of words in a language system.

Sensation: The conscious awareness of the arrival of the auditory signal.

Sensorineural hearing impairment: Often called a "nerve impairment," a sensorineural hearing impairment results from disease or damage located in the inner ear; usually a permanent hearing impairment.

Sensorineural mechanism: The part of the ear structure that includes the inner ear and acoustic nerve.

Sensory deprivation: Lack of auditory sensory input to the brain caused by a hearing impairment that can cause delayed and/or deviant behaviors.

Signal: Sounds that carry information to listeners.

Signal-to-noise (or Speech-to-Noise) ratio (S/N ratio): The relationship between the intensity of the signal of choice (in decibels), usually speech, and any sound (in decibels) that the person does not want to hear; a crucial concept for speech intelligibility.

Signal warning: The function of hearing that enables one to monitor the environment, including other people's interactions.

Sine wave: A periodic wave related to simple harmonic motion.

Site of lesion: The location in the auditory system where disease or damage occurs, causing hearing impairment.

Sound field: A space where sound is propagated.

Sound-field (classroom) FM amplification systems: Electronic equipment that amplifies an entire (class)room through the careful positioning of three to four wall- or ceiling-mounted loudspeakers; the teacher wears an FM microphone/transmitter.

Sound field testing: Calibrated auditory signals are presented through loudspeakers into the sound-isolated room rather than through headphones to test hearing; represented by the symbol "S" on an audiogram.

Sound-isolated room: An acoustically treated room where hearing tests should be performed to obtain accurate results.

Sound level: The intensity of sound in decibels.

Speech intelligibility: The percentage of the speech of a talker that is understood by a listener(s).

Speech-language pathologist: A specialist who has a graduate degree in speech and language disorders and how to alleviate them, and holds certification from the American Speech-Language-Hearing Association (ASHA).

Speech recognition or reception threshold (SRT): A test that determines the softest level that a person can just barely understand speech 50% of the time.

Speech sound improvement: Therapy directed at improving the production of specific sounds such as "r, s, l, sh, ch."

Static: Electrical discharges in a radio that cause crackling sounds and interfere with signal reception.

Stenosis: An abnormally small ear canal.

Stimulus: Something, such as a sound, that can evoke or elicit a response.

Support services: Ancillary services that are provided to assist a child in achieving academic success; services can include speech-language therapy, occupational therapy, aural habilitation, tutoring.

Suprasegmentals: Prosodic aspects of speech; variations in the pitch, loudness, rate, and duration of speech patterns.

Syndrome: A collection of anomalies that co-occur; hearing impairment often accompanies other disabilities or abnormalities, such as skeletal malformations or endocrine disorders.

Telecoil: A series of interconnected wire loops in a hearing aid that respond electrically to a magnetic signal.

Telecoil switch: An external control (switch) on a hearing aid that turns off the microphone and activates a telecoil in the hearing aid that picks up magnetic leakage from a telephone or the loop of an ALD; hearing aids for children need to come equipped with a telecoil.

Threshold: The intensity at which an individual can just barely hear a sound 50% of the time; all sounds louder than threshold can be heard, but softer sounds cannot be detected.

Tinnitus: Any of a number of internal head noises that can accompany hearing impairment; also called "ringing in the ears."

Tone control: A screw or knob for adjusting the frequency response of a sound system.

Transducer: A device such as a microphone or loudspeaker that changes sound into electricity (microphone) or changes electricity into sound (loudspeaker).

Transformer: A two-coil, induction device for increasing or decreasing the voltage of alternating current.

Transmitter: An apparatus that sends out electromagnetic rays; the FM system component that modulates the frequency of the radio signal in an audio frequency signal and sends the radio waves through the air to the antenna of the amplifier/receiver.

Trouble-shooting (hearing aids or ALDs): Performing various visual and listening inspections to determine whether an amplification unit is malfunctioning and, if so, evaluating the nature and severity of the malfunction.

Tuning fork tests: Part of a diagnostic audiologic assessment that involves a quick subjective screen of type and degree of hearing loss at the frequency (pitch) of the fork.

Tympanostomy tubes: Tiny ventilating tubes that are surgically inserted through the eardrum to replace a malfunctioning Eustachian tube in allowing ventilation of the middle ear space.

Unilateral hearing impairment: Hearing impairment in one ear; the other ear has normal hearing sensitivity. A unilateral hearing impairment can have a negative impact on a child's behavior, social skills, and development of spoken communication (language), due in large part to the reduction of incidental learning caused by the hearing loss.

Vent: A small hole or opening that serves as an outlet for sound in an earmold.

Vertigo: Dizziness that includes a sensation of spinning or whirling.

Vestibular system: Comprised of the saccule, utricle, and semicircular canals, the vestibular system is located in the inner ear and functions to regulate balance. Specifically, it coordinates changes in head position, acceleration and deceleration, and gravitational effects.

Vibrotactile: Pertains to the detection of vibrations through the sense of touch.

Vibrotactile hearing aid: An assistive listening device that converts acoustic energy into vibratory patterns that are delivered to the skin.

Visual reinforcement audiometry (VRA): A pediatric behavioral hearing test in which a child's auditory behaviors (usually localization) are conditioned to and rewarded by a visual display.

Voltmeter: An instrument that measures the number of volts between any two points in an electric circuit; used to test batteries when trouble-shooting amplification devices.

Volume control: A wheel or knob for adjusting the intensity of sound produced by a sound system.

Vowel: A speech sound identified by its unrestricted voice flow.

Wavelength: The distance between one peak of a sine wave and the next peak of the same wave.

Word discrimination testing (also called Word identification testing): Part of a diagnostic audiologic assessment where one determines how well words can be distinguished when they are presented at a typical conversational level of loudness and at an additional level loud enough to overcome the individual's hearing loss.

Wireless system: An FM transmitter and FM receiver; radio waves, not wires, connect the speaker and listener.

INDEX

■